The RN Pocket Guide: Nursing School Clinical Pocket Guide for Nursing Students

Natalie Spencer

Table of contents

Introduction: Your Clinical Confidence Starts Here....... 4

Chapter 1 — Preparing Before You Hit the Floor.......... 7

Chapter 2 — Vital Signs Done Right Every Time 13

Chapter 3 — Head-to-Toe Assessment Made Simple .. 21

Chapter 4 — Lab Values You Must Know 30

Chapter 5 — Medication Math and Safe Administration 40

Chapter 6 — IV Therapy and Fluid Essentials 50

Chapter 7 — Essential Clinical Procedures 61

Chapter 8 — Charting and Clinical Documentation..... 73

Chapter 9 — Emergencies and Rapid Response 85

Chapter 10 — Communication That Builds Trust........ 96

Conclusion: You Are Ready for the Bedside................ 106

Introduction: Your Clinical Confidence Starts Here

There is a moment every nursing student knows, even if nobody warned them about it. You have passed your exams. You can recite the stages of wound healing in your sleep. You have highlighted your pharmacology textbook until the pages glow. And then you walk onto a real hospital unit for the first time, wearing a badge that says *Student Nurse*, and everything you thought you knew seems to evaporate somewhere between the elevator and the nurses' station.

Your instructor turns to you and asks a simple question. "What did you notice about your patient's potassium this morning?" And your mind, which held that exact number twenty minutes ago, goes completely blank. Your patient's call light rings and you freeze for half a second, running through everything that could possibly be wrong before you even open the door. You watch the nurses around you move with an ease that feels impossible, and a quiet voice in the back of your head asks the question you would never say out loud: *Am I actually cut out for this?*

If any of that sounds familiar, take a breath. You are not behind. You are not failing. You are standing exactly where every nurse who came before you once stood, including the confident preceptor who seems to know everything. The gap you are feeling is not a gap in intelligence or dedication. It is the gap between classroom knowledge and bedside performance, and it is the single most predictable challenge of nursing school. Theory teaches you what to know. Clinical demands that you use it, in real time, with a real human being in front of you and an instructor watching over your shoulder. Nobody crosses that gap gracefully on the first try. But you can cross it faster, and with far less panic, when you have the right tool in your pocket.

That is exactly what this book is, and it is worth being clear about what it is not. This is not another textbook. You already own textbooks, and they are doing a fine job holding down your desk at home. They are built for depth, for studying, for two-hour reading sessions with coffee and a highlighter. They are not built for the hallway outside room 412 when you have ninety seconds to remember the normal range for a BUN, the steps of a focused respiratory assessment, or how to calculate a drip rate before your instructor arrives. This guide is built for precisely those moments. It lives in your scrub pocket. It is organized so you can flip to what you need in seconds, confirm your thinking, and get back to your patient. Every page earns its place by answering one question: will a student actually need this at the bedside? If the answer was no, it did not make the cut. What you are holding is the distilled, practical core of clinical practice, stripped of fluff and arranged for speed.

Here is how the journey unfolds. The book opens where every good shift opens: with preparation, showing you how to get organized before you ever touch the unit floor. From there it moves into the fundamentals you will perform on every single patient, starting with vital signs done accurately and interpreted intelligently, then building into the full head-to-toe assessment, broken down into a repeatable system you can trust. Next come the numbers that drive clinical decisions: the lab values you must know cold, what high and low results actually mean, and which ones demand immediate action. With assessment and labs in hand, the guide turns to medications, walking you through dosage calculations, safe administration, and the drug classes you will encounter daily, before extending into IV therapy, fluids, and electrolytes. Then it gets hands-on, covering the essential procedures students perform most, from catheters to wound care to drains. Because excellent care means nothing if it is not recorded, a full chapter is devoted to charting and documentation that protects both your patient and your license. The final stretch prepares you for the moments that test everyone: recognizing a deteriorating patient, knowing your role in an emergency, and communicating with patients, families, and providers in a way that builds real trust.

The order is deliberate. Each chapter stands on the one before it, the same way clinical competence actually develops, so you can read it front to back as a rotation companion or dive straight into whatever your shift throws at you. Tab the pages. Write in the margins. Let it get worn out, because a pristine pocket guide is a pocket guide that never got used.

You do not need to feel ready today. You need a reliable place to look when it counts, and the willingness to keep showing up. You bring the second part. The first part starts on the next page.

Chapter 1 — Preparing Before You Hit the Floor

1.1 The Night-Before Ritual That Changes Everything

Ask any clinical instructor to describe the difference between a student who thrives and a student who struggles, and most will tell you it has surprisingly little to do with GPA. The difference shows up before the shift ever starts. It shows up in whether the student walked onto the unit already knowing who their patient is, why that patient is in the hospital, and what the day is likely to demand — or whether they showed up hoping to figure it all out on the fly. Clinical performance is not born at the bedside. It is born the night before, at your kitchen table, in the thirty to sixty minutes you spend preparing while your classmates are telling themselves they will just wing it.

If your program gives you access to your patient assignment ahead of time, treat that access like gold. Start with the chart, but read it with a strategy instead of scrolling aimlessly. Your first stop is the admitting diagnosis and the history of present illness, because everything else in the chart only makes sense in that context. A potassium level means one thing in a healthy post-op patient and something very different in someone admitted with renal failure. Once you understand why the patient is there, move to the past medical history and build a quick mental picture of the whole person: their chronic conditions, their surgical history, anything that might complicate the primary problem. A patient admitted for pneumonia who also has heart failure and diabetes is really three clinical stories woven together, and you want to know all three before you introduce yourself.

From there, work through the pieces that will shape your actual shift. Scan the most recent provider notes and nursing notes to learn what has happened in the last twenty-four hours, because the patient you read about at 8 p.m. may have turned a corner — in either direction — by morning. Review the current medication list and flag anything unfamiliar. You do not need to memorize every drug tonight, but you should look up the ones you have never heard of, note why this patient is receiving them, and identify anything you would need to check before giving, such as a heart rate before a beta blocker or a blood pressure before an antihypertensive. Check the latest lab results and jot down anything outside normal range, then ask yourself the question your instructor will inevitably ask you: does this abnormal value make sense given the diagnosis, or is it something new? Finally, note the orders that will structure your day — diet, activity level, scheduled procedures, wound care, oxygen, telemetry, fluid restrictions. These small details are exactly what instructors quiz students on, precisely because they reveal whether you actually know your patient.

All of this information needs somewhere to live, and that somewhere should not be loose scraps of paper or your memory. This is where a personal clinical worksheet — often called a brain sheet — becomes your most valuable piece of equipment after your stethoscope. Nearly every working nurse uses some version of one. Yours can be a single page, organized however your mind works best, but it should have dedicated spaces for the essentials: patient initials and room number, code status, allergies, diagnosis and relevant history, abnormal labs, scheduled medications with their times, vital sign trends, assessment findings, and a running to-do list with checkboxes for tasks like dressing changes, blood glucose checks, and intake and output documentation. Fill in everything you can the night before. The blank spaces that remain become your morning agenda, which means you start the shift already knowing what you are looking for instead of reacting to whatever happens.

The morning of clinical deserves its own small ritual too. Get up early enough that nothing is rushed, because arriving flustered sets a tone that follows you all day. Eat something substantial — you may not sit down again for six or eight hours. Lay your uniform and supplies out the night before so the morning requires no decisions. On the drive or commute in, run through your patient's story once in your head, the way you would explain it to a friend: who they are, why they are here, what you are watching for. If you can summarize your patient in three or four sentences without looking at your sheet, you are prepared.

None of this takes talent. It takes about an hour of discipline the night before, repeated until it becomes automatic. Do it consistently and something remarkable happens: the anxiety that plagues most students begins to shrink, not because the clinical floor got easier, but because you stopped meeting it unprepared. Preparation is the quietest form of confidence, and it is entirely within your control.

1.2 Your Gear, Your Presence, and Your First Five Minutes

There is a particular sinking feeling that comes from reaching into your pocket for a penlight that is not there while your instructor waits for you to check pupillary response. Every item you carry is small, cheap, and utterly irreplaceable in the moment you need it, which is why your supplies deserve the same night-before attention as your patient chart. Your stethoscope comes first, and it should be a decent one, because a bargain-bin model that muffles lung sounds will sabotage assessments you are still learning to perform. Alongside it goes a penlight for neuro checks, a pair of bandage scissors, hemostats for clamping tubing or loosening stubborn caps, a permanent marker and pens in black ink, and a small notepad or your folded brain sheet on a clipboard. Add a watch with a second hand, since counting respirations by smartphone looks unprofessional and many units restrict phone use at the bedside anyway. Tuck in your pocket reference cards, this guide, and whatever your program requires you to have on your person, such as your student ID, and stock a few pairs of gloves in your size the moment you hit the floor. Assemble all of it the night before in the same pockets every time, so your hands learn where things live. A nurse who does not have to think about where the scissors are is a nurse whose mind is free for the patient.

How you look and carry yourself matters more than students want to believe, not because healthcare is a fashion contest but because patients decide within seconds whether they trust you. Arrive in a clean, wrinkle-free uniform that meets your program's dress code exactly, with closed-toe shoes, hair secured away from your face, nails short and unpolished, and jewelry minimal. Perfume and cologne stay home, since scents can trigger nausea in patients who are already miserable. Just as important is what your conduct communicates: put the phone away, do not chew gum, stand when someone needs help rather than watching from the nurses' station, and never discuss patients in elevators, hallways, or the cafeteria. Confidentiality violations end nursing school careers, and the walls of a hospital genuinely do have ears.

Then comes the moment that intimidates students most: introducing yourself. Walk up to the nurse you are assigned to, make eye contact, and keep it simple. Give your name, your school, your level in the program, and what you are able to do today, then ask what would be most helpful. Something like, "Hi, I'm Sam, a second-semester nursing student. I can do full assessments, vital signs, and med passes with my instructor. What would you like me to jump in on?" tells a busy nurse exactly how to use you, and nurses respect students who make their role clear. Learn the names of the charge nurse and the aides, thank people who teach you something, and if a nurse seems short with you, do not take it personally — she may be three admissions deep. Offer to help with the unglamorous work, because answering call lights and fetching warm blankets buys you more goodwill and learning opportunities than any credential.

1.3 Setting Goals So Clinical Works for You

Most students walk into clinical with one unspoken goal: survive until post-conference. That is understandable, but it quietly wastes the most expensive education you will ever pay for. Every clinical day is a limited resource, and students who extract the most from it share one habit: they arrive with specific, stated learning goals instead of waiting to be assigned tasks.

The framework is straightforward. Start with your course objectives, which your syllabus lists for a reason — your instructor is evaluating you against them, so aligning your goals with them makes you easier to teach and easier to grade well. Then make each goal concrete enough that you will know by end of shift whether you met it. "Get better at assessments" is a wish. "Complete a full head-to-toe on my patient before 0900 and have my instructor verify my lung sounds" is a goal. Aim for two or three per shift, mixing one skill you have never done, one skill you need to repeat for confidence, and one knowledge goal, such as being able to explain every medication you administer. Tie at least one goal to your specific patient, because a goal like "understand how heart failure changes my assessment priorities" turns an ordinary shift into a case study.

Now say your goals out loud. At the start of the shift, tell your instructor directly: "Today I'd like to attempt my first Foley insertion if one comes up, and I want you to check my documentation before I submit it." This one habit transforms your clinical experience, because instructors funnel opportunities toward students who ask for them. If a catheter insertion comes up on the other side of the unit, the instructor now knows to come find you. At the end of the shift, close the loop by briefly reviewing what you met, what you missed, and what carries over to next week. That five-minute reflection is where experience actually converts into learning.

This shift — from passenger to pilot of your own education — is the real lesson of this chapter. Preparation gets you to the floor ready; goals make the floor work for you. With both habits in place, you are ready for the clinical skills themselves, beginning with the one you will perform more than any other: vital signs.

Chapter 2 — Vital Signs Done Right Every Time

2.1 The Six Measurements You Will Take Thousands of Times

Vital signs are the first clinical skill most students learn, which is exactly why so many students stop taking them seriously. They feel routine. They feel like a task to finish before the real nursing begins. Then one day a patient's blood pressure reads 82/50, and suddenly the "routine" task is the entire story of the shift. Vital signs are the earliest warning system medicine has, and the nurse who takes them carelessly is a nurse flying with the instrument panel switched off. Learn to take them correctly now, while someone is still watching over your shoulder, and accuracy will be your habit for the next forty years.

Start with blood pressure, because it is the measurement students get wrong most often. Position matters before the cuff ever inflates: the patient should be seated or lying with the arm supported at heart level, legs uncrossed, and ideally resting quietly for a few minutes beforehand. An arm dangling below the heart can read falsely high; an arm propped above it reads falsely low. Cuff size is the next trap. A cuff too small for the arm produces a falsely elevated reading, while an oversized cuff underestimates, so check that the bladder wraps around roughly eighty percent of the arm's circumference. Place the cuff on bare skin, not over a sleeve, with its lower edge about an inch above the antecubital fossa and the artery marker aligned over the brachial artery. If you are taking a manual pressure, palpate the radial pulse while inflating, note where it disappears, inflate about thirty more millimeters of mercury beyond that point, then deflate slowly — around two to three millimeters per second — listening for the first Korotkoff sound (systolic) and the point where sounds vanish (diastolic). Deflating too fast is the classic student error, and it chops accuracy off both numbers. Never take a pressure on an arm with an IV line, a dialysis fistula, lymphedema, or on the same side as a mastectomy. If a reading surprises you, wait a minute or two and repeat it yourself, on the other arm if appropriate, before you chart or report it.

Heart rate comes next, and the rule that protects you is simple: fingers, not thumb. Your thumb has a pulse of its own and will happily lie to you. Press two fingers over the radial artery, and if the rhythm is regular, counting for thirty seconds and doubling is acceptable. The moment the rhythm feels irregular, count for a full sixty seconds, and for any patient with a cardiac history or on rhythm-affecting medications like digoxin or beta blockers, take an apical pulse with your stethoscope at the fifth intercostal space, midclavicular line, for a full minute. While you count, pay attention to more than the number — strength and regularity are findings too, and "irregularly irregular" is a phrase that should always reach the provider.

Respiratory rate is the most falsified vital sign in healthcare, usually recorded as a reflexive "16" without anyone actually counting. Do not inherit that habit. The challenge is that patients who know you are watching their breathing change it, so use the old trick: keep your fingers on the radial pulse after you finish counting the heart rate and count respirations while the patient believes you are still checking their pulse. Count for thirty seconds and double, or a full minute if breathing is irregular, shallow, or labored. Note depth and effort, not just rate, because a rate of 22 with accessory muscle use is a very different patient than a rate of 22 chatting comfortably.

Temperature is more straightforward, but route matters and must be charted. Oral readings require the probe in the sublingual pocket with lips closed, and they are unreliable if the patient just drank something hot or cold — wait fifteen minutes. Tympanic thermometers need a gentle ear pull up and back in adults to straighten the canal. Temporal scanners must actually contact the skin and sweep across the forehead; sweat and hair throw them off. Axillary readings run roughly half a degree to a full degree lower than oral and are a last resort in adults. Whatever route you use, record it, because a rectal 38.0 and an axillary 38.0 are not the same fever.

Oxygen saturation seems foolproof — clip and read — which is precisely why it fools people. Cold fingers, nail polish, artificial nails, poor perfusion, tremors, and ambient light all corrupt the number. If the reading seems wrong, warm the hand, try another finger or an earlobe probe, and confirm the pulse the device displays matches the pulse you palpate; if those two numbers disagree, the saturation cannot be trusted. Always chart whether the patient is on room air or supplemental oxygen, and how much, because a saturation of 95 percent means something entirely different on four liters than on none.

Finally, pain — the vital sign with no machine. Ask, using a zero-to-ten scale, and accept the patient's answer as data even when their face disagrees, while still documenting objective signs like grimacing or guarding. Ask about location, quality, and what makes it better or worse. For patients who cannot self-report, use the behavioral scale your facility designates rather than guessing.

Across all six, one habit separates safe students from risky ones: when a value is abnormal or unexpected, recheck it yourself before acting on it or dismissing it — and if it holds, report it. A recheck takes ninety seconds. A missed trend can take much more.

2.2 Knowing What Normal Looks Like So You Can Spot What Doesn't

Numbers mean nothing without a frame around them. Collecting vital signs is a mechanical skill; interpreting them is a clinical one, and interpretation begins with knowing what you expect to see in a healthy body. For the average adult, a resting heart rate falls between 60 and 100 beats per minute. Blood pressure sits below 120/80 in an ideal reading, with anything above 130/80 now classified as hypertension and anything below 90/60 raising the concern of hypotension. Respiratory rate in a calm, resting adult is 12 to 20 breaths per minute. Oral temperature ranges from about 36.1 to 37.2 degrees Celsius, or roughly 97.0 to 99.0 degrees Fahrenheit. Oxygen saturation should be 95 percent or above on room air in most patients, though your patients with chronic obstructive pulmonary disease may live comfortably at 88 to 92 percent, and their providers will have set individualized targets. Memorize these numbers the way you know your own phone number, because every clinical judgment you make starts by comparing what you measured to what you expected.

Those ranges shift at the edges of life. Pediatric patients run faster and smaller: a newborn's heart rate can sit between 120 and 160 beats per minute and a respiratory rate of 30 to 60 is entirely normal, numbers that would trigger alarms in an adult. Blood pressure in children is lower, and you will need age- and height-based percentile charts rather than a single cutoff. Toddlers and infants also spike fevers more dramatically and desaturate faster because their oxygen reserves are smaller, which means the window between "worth watching" and "needs intervention now" is narrower. On the other end of the spectrum, elderly patients bring their own variations. Baseline blood pressure often runs higher due to arterial stiffness, resting heart rate may sit lower if they are on rate-controlling medications, and temperature response can be blunted — an older adult with a serious infection may never mount a fever at all, which makes other signs like confusion, tachycardia, or falling blood pressure even more important to catch.

Knowing the ranges is step one. Step two is asking yourself what an abnormal value is trying to tell you. A heart rate above 100 — tachycardia — is not a diagnosis; it is a signal, and the list of things driving it ranges from anxiety and pain to dehydration, blood loss, fever, and cardiac arrhythmia. Your job is not to diagnose the cause, but to pair the number with everything else you see. A tachycardic patient who is also hypotensive and pale tells a very different story than a tachycardic patient who just walked back from physical therapy. Hypotension — a systolic below 90 or a drop of 20 or more from the patient's baseline — should always sharpen your attention, because it can reflect hemorrhage, sepsis, cardiac failure, medication side effects, or severe dehydration, all of which deteriorate quickly. Fever above 38.3 degrees Celsius in a hospitalized patient demands investigation: new infection, surgical site complication, drug reaction, or blood product response are all on the table, and the provider will want to know. Desaturation below 90 percent on room air or below a patient's established target is an urgent finding that calls for immediate assessment of airway, breathing, and level of consciousness before anything else.

The key question to develop as a habit is not just "is this number abnormal?" but "is this number new, and is it changing?" A blood pressure of 100/60 in a patient who has been running 100/62 all week is a baseline. The same reading in someone whose pressure was 138/82 two hours ago is a warning. Trend matters more than any isolated number, which is why charting accurately and reviewing prior values before you take your own set is so important.

2.3 The Vital Sign Skills That Set You Apart

Once you can measure and interpret a standard set of vitals, there are a few deeper techniques that separate competent students from impressive ones. The first is orthostatic vital signs, sometimes called tilt testing, used to evaluate whether a patient's cardiovascular system is compensating adequately for position changes. The procedure is straightforward: take a blood pressure and heart rate with the patient lying flat, then repeat both after the patient has been sitting upright for one to two minutes, and finally repeat again after standing for one to two minutes. A systolic drop of 20 millimeters of mercury or more, a diastolic drop of 10 or more, or a heart rate increase of 20 or more beats per minute between positions qualifies as a positive orthostatic finding and suggests volume depletion or autonomic dysfunction. This is not an exotic skill — it is deeply practical on any medical-surgical floor where patients are post-operative, on diuretics, have been vomiting, or are simply elderly and at risk for falls. When you chart orthostatics, always document the patient's position and the time of each measurement, not just the numbers, because two minutes of standing produces a more reliable reading than ten seconds.

Mean arterial pressure — MAP — is the next concept worth understanding early. You will see it on monitor screens and in provider orders, and the formula is not difficult: add one-third of the systolic to two-thirds of the diastolic, or use the shortcut of diastolic plus one-third of the pulse pressure. A MAP of 65 or above is generally considered the minimum needed to perfuse vital organs. When a patient's MAP drops below that threshold, you are looking at a perfusion problem that requires prompt communication, because kidneys, brain, and heart are not receiving adequate blood flow. Many ICU and step-down orders include MAP targets for titrating vasopressors, and even on a general floor, calculating MAP from a manual pressure gives you a faster read on hemodynamic status than the two numbers alone.

Pulse pressure deserves attention too, though students rarely think about it. It is simply the difference between systolic and diastolic. Normal pulse pressure runs roughly 40 millimeters of mercury. A widened pulse pressure — say, 160/60 — can suggest aortic regurgitation, increased intracranial pressure, or hyperthyroidism. A narrowed pulse pressure — say, 90/74 — hints at reduced cardiac output, tension pneumothorax, or significant blood loss, because the heart is struggling to generate enough force to separate those two numbers. Neither finding alone makes a diagnosis, but combined with your other assessment data, it adds a layer of clinical reasoning that most students have not yet developed, and instructors notice.

All of these skills converge into one critical nursing behavior: recognizing when a vital sign change demands a phone call to the provider. In general, you should pick up the phone whenever a systolic pressure drops below 90 or rises above 180, when heart rate falls below 50 or exceeds 130, when respiratory rate drops below 8 or rises above 28, when oxygen saturation falls below 90 percent despite intervention, when temperature exceeds 38.5 degrees Celsius in a vulnerable patient, when MAP falls below 65, or when orthostatic measurements are positive in a symptomatic patient — meaning they are dizzy, lightheaded, or near-syncopal on standing. When you do call, use the SBAR framework your program has taught you: state the situation, give background, share your assessment including the specific numbers and how they have changed, and make a recommendation or request. Providers respect nurses who bring data, not just worry, and as a student, showing that you can pair a concerning number with context and a clear request is one of the fastest ways to earn trust from your clinical team.

Vital signs are the foundation everything else sits on. You will take them countless times across your career, and it would be easy to let them feel routine. Resist that. The day you stop paying attention to the numbers is the day you miss the one that matters most.

Chapter 3 — Head-to-Toe Assessment Made Simple

3.1 One System at a Time, Every Patient, Every Shift

The head-to-toe assessment is the skill that separates someone who checks on patients from someone who actually assesses them. It is also the skill that terrifies students most, largely because nursing school presents it as an overwhelming marathon of inspection, palpation, percussion, and auscultation across every square inch of the human body, all performed flawlessly in under twenty minutes while your instructor silently grades you. In practice, the full assessment becomes manageable the moment you stop thinking of it as a single enormous task and start treating it as a series of small, predictable steps organized by body system. The framework below works the same way whether your patient is a 34-year-old post-appendectomy or a 78-year-old with heart failure. Learn the sequence once, repeat it until it becomes automatic, and you will never again stand at the bedside wondering where to begin.

Start at the top, literally, with a neurological check. Before you lay a hand on the patient, you are already assessing: are they awake, alert, and oriented? Ask them to tell you their name, where they are, and the approximate date. That gives you orientation to person, place, and time, the basic three. Note their speech — is it clear and coherent, or slurred and confused? Observe their facial symmetry as they talk; a droop on one side warrants immediate escalation. Check pupil size and reactivity with your penlight, comparing both sides — pupils should be equal, round, and reactive to light. Test grip strength bilaterally by having the patient squeeze two of your fingers, then ask them to push and pull their feet against your hands to assess lower extremity strength. Any new-onset weakness, asymmetry, or change from the patient's baseline is a finding that cannot wait.

Move to the head, eyes, ears, nose, and throat. Inspect the scalp for lesions or tenderness if relevant, examine the conjunctiva of the eyes by gently pulling down the lower lid — pale conjunctiva can suggest anemia. Check the mucous membranes of the mouth for moisture, color, and integrity; dry, cracked lips and a sticky tongue point toward dehydration, while white patches could signal a fungal infection. Note the condition of the teeth or dentures, since oral health directly affects nutrition and infection risk. If the patient has a nasogastric tube or endotracheal tube, inspect the insertion site and surrounding tissue for irritation or breakdown while you are in the area.

The respiratory assessment comes next and deserves your full attention because it reveals problems faster than almost any lab value. Observe the patient's breathing before you touch the chest: count the rate, watch for use of accessory muscles in the neck and shoulders, and note whether the patient can speak in full sentences or has to pause for breath. Then listen. Place your stethoscope on bare skin — listening through a hospital gown muffles sounds and creates artifact — and auscultate systematically, side to side, starting at the apices above the clavicles and working down through six to eight posterior fields. You are listening for air movement that is equal bilaterally and clear. Crackles, especially at the bases, may suggest fluid; wheezes suggest bronchospasm or narrowed airways; diminished or absent sounds over one area demand immediate follow-up. If the patient has a cough, note whether it is dry or productive, and if productive, the color and consistency of the sputum. Always document the oxygen delivery device and flow rate alongside your findings.

The cardiovascular assessment follows naturally. Inspect the neck for jugular venous distension with the patient reclined at about 45 degrees — visible, bounding jugular veins can indicate fluid overload or right-sided heart failure. Auscultate heart sounds at the four classic valve sites: aortic at the right second intercostal space, pulmonic at the left second intercostal space, tricuspid at the left lower sternal border, and mitral at the fifth intercostal space midclavicular line. Listen for rate, rhythm, and any extra sounds — a new murmur, a gallop rhythm like an S3 or S4, or a pericardial rub are all findings to report. Palpate peripheral pulses bilaterally — radial, dorsalis pedis, and posterior tibial — and compare strength. Inspect the lower extremities for edema by pressing your thumb firmly over the shin or medial malleolus for a few seconds; if the indentation remains, grade it from one-plus to four-plus and measure how far up the leg it extends. Check capillary refill by pressing a fingernail bed and releasing — color should return in under three seconds.

Now move to the abdomen. Have the patient lie flat if possible and inspect first: note shape, distension, symmetry, and any visible scars, tubes, or ostomies. Here is the one place where the usual order changes — auscultate before you palpate or percuss, because touching the abdomen can alter bowel sounds. Listen in all four quadrants with the diaphragm of your stethoscope. Normal bowel sounds are irregular gurgling clicks, occurring roughly five to thirty times per minute. Absent sounds require listening for at least two full minutes in each quadrant before you call them absent, and hyperactive or high-pitched tinkling sounds may suggest an obstruction or gastroenteritis. After auscultating, lightly palpate all four quadrants, watching the patient's face for grimacing rather than relying on them to tell you it hurts, since many patients minimize discomfort. Note any rigidity, guarding, masses, or tenderness. If the patient has a surgical incision, assess the dressing or wound for drainage, approximation, and signs of infection — redness, warmth, swelling, or purulent discharge.

The musculoskeletal and integumentary assessment wraps things up. Observe the patient's ability to move all four extremities and change position. Check the skin systematically, paying special attention to pressure-prone areas: the sacrum, heels, elbows, and the back of the head in patients with limited mobility. Look for redness that does not blanch when pressed, because non-blanchable erythema is a Stage 1 pressure injury and needs to be documented and reported immediately. Note any bruising, skin tears, rashes, or changes in skin color. Inspect intravenous sites for redness, swelling, or tenderness that could indicate phlebitis or infiltration. For patients with devices — urinary catheters, drains, wound vacs — include those in your sweep, checking that everything is patent, secured, and functioning.

The entire sequence, once practiced, takes twelve to fifteen minutes and follows a head-to-heels path that keeps you from skipping systems or doubling back. The secret is consistency: do it the same way every time, on every patient, so the normal findings become so familiar that the abnormal ones practically announce themselves. You are not searching for disease. You are getting to know what your patient looks and sounds like right now, so that when something changes three hours later, you catch it — because you knew what came before.

3.2 When You Don't Need the Whole Picture — Focused Assessments That Save Time and Catch Trouble

A full head-to-toe assessment is essential at the start of every shift, but you will not repeat the entire sequence every time you walk into your patient's room. Between your initial assessment and the end of the shift, you will check on your patient multiple times, and each of those encounters calls for a focused assessment — a targeted evaluation of the body system or systems most relevant to the patient's diagnosis, complaint, or change in condition. Knowing when to narrow your scope and what to zero in on is one of the clearest markers that a student is developing real clinical judgment rather than mechanically repeating a checklist.

A focused cardiac assessment is appropriate any time you are caring for a patient with a cardiac history, chest pain, new arrhythmias, or hemodynamic changes. Start by asking the patient directly: do you have any chest pain, pressure, or tightness right now? Any shortness of breath, dizziness, or palpitations? Then assess: auscultate heart sounds at the four valve sites, listening for rate, rhythm, and any new murmur or extra sound that was not present during your earlier assessment. Check the blood pressure and compare it to the prior reading. Inspect the neck for jugular venous distension. Palpate pedal pulses bilaterally and note any new or worsening edema in the lower extremities. Check capillary refill. Look at the cardiac monitor if the patient is on telemetry — know the rhythm, know the rate, and know whether it has changed. Red flags that demand immediate escalation include new-onset chest pain, a systolic pressure below 90 or above 180, a heart rate below 50 or above 150, new irregular rhythms, absent peripheral pulses, and oxygen desaturation accompanying any cardiac symptom.

A focused respiratory assessment is your go-to for any patient admitted with pneumonia, COPD exacerbation, asthma, pulmonary embolism, or post-operative respiratory compromise. Ask whether the patient feels short of breath, whether their breathing is better or worse than the last time you checked, and whether they have a new or worsening cough. Observe their work of breathing before you reach for the stethoscope — accessory muscle use, nasal flaring, tripod positioning, and inability to speak in full sentences tell you the severity before you hear a single lung sound. Auscultate all lung fields, comparing side to side, and note whether sounds that were previously clear have developed crackles, wheezes, or diminished air movement. Check the oxygen saturation and the current delivery device. Red flags here include a respiratory rate below 10 or above 28, saturation falling below 90 percent despite supplemental oxygen, sudden onset of dyspnea, audible stridor, or asymmetric chest expansion, which can suggest pneumothorax.

For an abdominal focused assessment, think of patients with GI diagnoses, post-surgical abdomens, nausea and vomiting, or complaints of new pain. Ask about the last bowel movement, the presence of gas, any nausea, and whether the pain is constant or comes and goes. Ask them to point to where it hurts rather than suggesting a location, because leading the patient introduces bias. Auscultate bowel sounds in all four quadrants before palpating. Lightly palpate away from the painful area first, working toward it, watching the patient's face the entire time. Inspect any surgical sites, drains, or ostomies for output and integrity. Red flags include a rigid, board-like abdomen, rebound tenderness, absent bowel sounds after adequate listening time, new abdominal distension, bloody or coffee-ground emesis, and significant changes in drain output color or volume.

A focused neurological assessment applies to patients with stroke, seizure history, traumatic brain injury, altered mental status, or those recovering from neurological procedures. Assess orientation, speech clarity, facial symmetry, pupil reactivity and equality, and bilateral grip strength and foot push-pull — the same quick battery from your head-to-toe, but now you are comparing results to a known baseline from earlier in the shift. Ask the patient if they have a headache, vision changes, numbness, or tingling. Red flags include any new asymmetry in strength or facial movement, pupil inequality, sudden confusion, slurred speech, severe headache, or a decline in level of consciousness. These findings cannot wait for the next scheduled assessment — they need to reach the provider immediately.

Musculoskeletal focused assessments come into play for patients recovering from joint replacements, fractures, falls, or spinal procedures. Assess the affected extremity for range of motion within ordered restrictions, sensation, circulation distal to the injury or surgical site, and pain level with movement. Compare warmth, color, and swelling to the opposite limb. For post-surgical patients with casts or splints, check for the five P's: pain, pallor, pulselessness, paresthesia, and paralysis, any one of which could indicate compartment syndrome and qualifies as an emergency.

The common thread across every focused assessment is intentionality. You are not simply popping in to "see how they're doing." You are walking in with a question — is this system stable, improving, or declining? — and walking out with an answer you can chart and, if needed, communicate.

3.3 Saying What You Found in the Language the Chart Demands

There is a frustrating gap between knowing what you observed and writing it down in a way that sounds like a nurse wrote it. Every student has stood in front of a computer screen knowing exactly what their patient's lungs sounded like but typing something clumsy like "lungs sound fine" or "breathing OK" because the professional phrasing would not come. The distance between a casual observation and proper clinical documentation is not intelligence — it is vocabulary, and vocabulary is learned fastest through examples.

Normal findings have standard language that you will see repeated across charts in every hospital in the country, and the sooner it becomes your default, the more confident your documentation will look. When lung sounds are normal, the charting phrase is "bilateral lung sounds clear to auscultation in all fields." When heart sounds are normal, you write "heart sounds S1 and S2 auscultated, regular rate and rhythm, no murmur, rub, or gallop noted." A normal abdominal assessment reads something like "abdomen soft, non-tender, non-distended, bowel sounds present and normoactive in all four quadrants." For a neurological baseline, "patient alert and oriented to person, place, and time; speech clear; pupils equal, round, and reactive to light; bilateral grip strength and lower extremity strength equal and strong." Skin documentation follows the pattern of "skin warm, dry, and intact; no rashes, lesions, or areas of breakdown noted; IV site in right forearm without redness, swelling, or tenderness." Peripheral vascular findings chart as "bilateral pedal pulses palpable and equal; capillary refill less than three seconds; no edema noted in lower extremities."

Abnormal findings require more precision, because vague documentation fails the next nurse, the provider, and potentially the patient. Instead of writing "some swelling in legs," you write "two-plus pitting edema noted bilaterally to mid-shin." Instead of "patient seems confused," you write "patient oriented to person only; unable to state location or date; speech tangential." Rather than "wound looks infected," you document "surgical incision to right lower quadrant with surrounding erythema extending approximately two centimeters from wound edge; moderate amount of yellow-green purulent drainage on gauze dressing; wound edges approximated with staples intact; area warm to palpation." The difference is specificity: size, location, color, quantity, and comparison to prior findings. When describing pain, document the patient's self-reported score, location, quality, and what you observed — "patient rates pain at seven out of ten, described as sharp and constant in right upper quadrant; patient observed guarding and grimacing with palpation."

A few documentation principles save students from common mistakes. Always chart what you actually assessed, not what you assumed. If you did not listen to bowel sounds, do not write that they were normoactive. Use objective language and avoid subjective interpretations; "patient appears anxious" is acceptable, but "patient is overreacting" is not — and it can become a legal liability. Avoid the word "normal" on its own; specify what normal means in measurable terms so anyone reading the chart at three in the morning knows exactly what you found. Chart in real time whenever possible, because recreating your findings from memory two hours later introduces errors and omissions. And when in doubt about how to phrase something, look at how experienced nurses have charted similar findings on the same patient — the chart itself is one of the best teaching tools available to you.

Building this vocabulary takes practice, but it does not take long. Within a few shifts of deliberately using proper terminology, these phrases will come automatically, and your documentation will read like that of a nurse who has been doing this for years rather than a student still finding the words. The bridge between your assessment skills and your charting skills is where clinical credibility lives, and the documentation chapter later in this book will build on the foundation you are setting right now.

Chapter 4 — Lab Values You Must Know

4.1 The Numbers Behind Every Clinical Decision

There will come a morning, probably sooner than you expect, when your instructor rounds on you and asks a deceptively simple question: "What are your patient's labs today?" In that moment, you will either know the answer or you will not, and there is no middle ground that looks good. Lab values drive nearly every major decision in the hospital — whether to give a medication, hold it, call the provider, adjust fluids, order imaging, or discharge the patient — and the nurse is almost always the first person to see the results come through. If you cannot interpret the basics, you are relying on someone else to catch what you missed. This section organizes the labs you will encounter most often into categories you can scan in seconds, because speed matters when you are looking something up between a med pass and an assessment.

Start with the complete blood count, the CBC, because it is ordered on virtually every patient who walks through the door. White blood cells are your infection and immunity marker, with a normal range generally falling between 4,500 and 11,000 cells per microliter. An elevated white count — leukocytosis — suggests the body is fighting something: infection, inflammation, stress response, or occasionally leukemia. A depressed white count — leukopenia — raises concern for bone marrow suppression, which you will see in patients on chemotherapy, certain immunosuppressants, or those with overwhelming sepsis that has exhausted the marrow's reserves. Hemoglobin and hematocrit tell you about oxygen-carrying capacity. Normal hemoglobin runs roughly 12 to 16 grams per deciliter for women and 14 to 18 for men, while hematocrit, the percentage of blood volume occupied by red cells, tracks at about three times the hemoglobin value. Low values indicate anemia from blood loss, chronic disease, iron deficiency, or nutritional deficit; high values can appear with dehydration, polycythemia, or chronic hypoxia as the body compensates by producing more red cells. Platelets round out the CBC, normally between 150,000 and 400,000 per microliter. Low platelets — thrombocytopenia — put the patient at risk for bleeding and can result from heparin therapy, liver disease, chemotherapy, or autoimmune destruction. Elevated platelets may signal inflammation, infection, or a myeloproliferative disorder, and they increase clotting risk.

The basic metabolic panel, or BMP, gives you a snapshot of electrolytes, kidney function, and blood sugar. Sodium normally runs 136 to 145 milliequivalents per liter. Low sodium — hyponatremia — is one of the most common electrolyte imbalances in hospitalized patients and can be caused by fluid overload, diuretics, SIADH, or excessive free water intake; symptoms include confusion, lethargy, and in severe cases, seizures. High sodium — hypernatremia — usually signals dehydration or inadequate free water. Potassium is arguably the most dangerous electrolyte to get wrong, with a narrow normal range of 3.5 to 5.0 milliequivalents per liter. Hypokalemia can be triggered by diuretics, vomiting, NG suction, or poor intake, and it puts the heart at risk for dangerous arrhythmias. Hyperkalemia, often seen in renal failure, crush injuries, or with potassium-sparing diuretics and ACE inhibitors, carries its own cardiac risks, including peaked T-waves on the ECG and potentially fatal ventricular arrhythmias. Blood urea nitrogen, or BUN, normally falls between 7 and 20 milligrams per deciliter, and creatinine sits between 0.6 and 1.2 milligrams per deciliter; together they assess how well the kidneys are filtering waste. Elevated values suggest renal impairment, dehydration, or high protein catabolism, and they directly affect medication dosing for drugs cleared by the kidneys. Glucose on the BMP should range from 70 to 100 milligrams per deciliter fasting, and you will watch it closely in diabetic patients, patients on corticosteroids, patients receiving TPN, and anyone who is NPO but still receiving insulin or oral hypoglycemics.

The comprehensive metabolic panel, or CMP, includes everything in the BMP plus liver function markers and additional proteins. Albumin, normally 3.5 to 5.0 grams per deciliter, reflects nutritional status and liver synthetic function; a low albumin is common in malnourished, critically ill, or liver failure patients and affects wound healing, fluid distribution, and drug binding. Total protein, ranging from 6.0 to 8.3 grams per deciliter, provides a broader picture of the same. The liver enzymes — AST and ALT — normally fall below about 35 to 40 international units per liter depending on the lab, and elevations point to hepatocellular damage from hepatitis, drug toxicity (acetaminophen being the classic culprit), alcohol use, or ischemia. Alkaline phosphatase, normally 44 to 147 international units per liter, rises with biliary obstruction, bone disease, or liver pathology. Bilirubin, both total and direct, rounds out the liver picture; total bilirubin normally stays below 1.2 milligrams per deciliter, and elevations produce the visible jaundice you may notice during your skin assessment, pointing to liver dysfunction, hemolysis, or bile duct obstruction.

The coagulation panel becomes essential the moment your patient is on any blood-thinning therapy. Prothrombin time, or PT, normally runs 11 to 13.5 seconds, and the INR — the standardized ratio derived from it — is 1.0 in a healthy person. Patients on warfarin typically have a therapeutic INR target of 2.0 to 3.0, though mechanical heart valve patients may need 2.5 to 3.5. An INR above the therapeutic range puts the patient at serious bleeding risk; below it means inadequate anticoagulation. Partial thromboplastin time, or PTT, normally falls between 25 and 35 seconds and monitors heparin therapy. An aPTT that runs too high means too much heparin and bleeding danger; too low means the clot risk you are trying to prevent is still present. Ddimer is a degradation product of fibrin and rises when the body is breaking down clots; it is commonly used in the emergency setting to help evaluate for deep vein thrombosis or pulmonary embolism, with a normal value below 500 nanograms per milliliter in most labs.

Cardiac markers come into focus whenever chest pain or a suspected cardiac event enters the picture. Troponin is the gold standard for myocardial injury, with most labs setting the upper limit of normal below 0.04 nanograms per milliliter, though high-sensitivity troponin assays use even lower cutoffs. Troponin rises within a few hours of heart muscle damage and can remain elevated for up to two weeks, making it both sensitive and persistent. B-type natriuretic peptide, or BNP, is released when the heart's ventricles are stretched by volume overload, and levels above 100 picograms per milliliter raise suspicion for heart failure, with higher numbers correlating to greater severity. Creatine kinase and its MB fraction — CK and CK-MB — are older cardiac markers that have largely been supplemented by troponin but may still appear in your patient's labs, particularly as a trend to evaluate timing and extent of injury.

Finally, urinalysis gives you a window into renal function, hydration, infection, and metabolic status without drawing a single drop of blood. Normal urine is clear to slightly yellow, with a specific gravity between 1.005 and 1.030 reflecting concentration. The presence of leukocyte esterase and nitrites suggests a urinary tract infection and warrants a culture. Protein in the urine may indicate kidney damage, while glucose spilling into urine points to blood sugars high enough to exceed the renal threshold, commonly seen in uncontrolled diabetes. Red blood cells in the urine can originate anywhere from the kidneys to the urethra, and ketones appear during diabetic ketoacidosis, starvation, or prolonged vomiting.

None of these values exist in isolation. A low potassium means more when you know the patient is on furosemide. An elevated troponin means more when you know they came in with chest pain. The real skill is connecting the number to the patient lying in front of you, and that connection is what the rest of this chapter will build.

4.2 When a Lab Value Cannot Wait — Critical Results and Your Legal Obligation

Most lab results arrive quietly. They populate the chart, you review them during your assessment, and you incorporate them into your plan of care. But certain values fall so far outside normal range that they represent an immediate threat to the patient's life, and the moment one of those results appears, a clock starts ticking — not a figurative one, but a very real regulatory and legal one. These are called critical values, sometimes referred to as panic values, and every hospital maintains a specific list defining which results qualify and at what thresholds. The laboratory is required to notify the nursing staff directly when a critical value is resulted, usually by phone, and from that moment forward, the responsibility for acting on it belongs to you.

The thresholds vary slightly between institutions, but the values that appear on nearly every critical list are consistent enough that you should commit them to memory. A potassium below 3.0 or above 6.0 milliequivalents per liter is critical because of the immediate risk of fatal cardiac arrhythmia. Sodium below 120 or above 160 milliequivalents per liter can produce seizures, coma, and death. Glucose below 40 milligrams per deciliter represents severe hypoglycemia with risk of loss of consciousness and brain injury; above 500 milligrams per deciliter, the patient may be in or approaching diabetic ketoacidosis or hyperosmolar hyperglycemic state. A hemoglobin below 7.0 grams per deciliter often triggers a transfusion conversation, and a platelet count below 50,000 per microliter puts the patient at significant spontaneous bleeding risk, with counts below 20,000 creating a near-emergency. An INR above 5.0 in a patient on warfarin carries serious hemorrhage potential. Troponin elevations above the institution's critical threshold signal acute myocardial injury. A white blood cell count below 2,000 suggests profound immunosuppression, and a calcium below 6.5 or above 13.0 milligrams per deciliter threatens cardiac and neuromuscular function. These are not numbers to memorize for an exam and then forget — they are numbers that, if you miss them or delay acting on them, can directly cause patient harm.

Your responsibility when a critical value is called to you follows a clear four-step sequence: verify, notify, document, and reassess. Verification means confirming that the result belongs to your patient and that the specimen was collected properly. Lab errors happen. Hemolyzed samples can falsely elevate potassium. A blood draw from an arm with a running IV can dilute results and produce falsely low values. If the result does not match the clinical picture at all — a potassium of 6.8 in a patient who was 4.2 this morning with no renal issues — it is reasonable to ask the lab to re-run the specimen or to collect a fresh one, but you must still notify the provider of the initial result while that process is underway. Never sit on a critical value waiting for a redraw to come back. Notification means calling the provider directly, not sending a message through the electronic chart and hoping someone reads it. Use SBAR to structure the call: state which patient, the critical result, what the prior value was if you have it, the patient's current clinical status, and what you are requesting — new orders, a repeat lab, a bedside evaluation, whatever the situation demands. Document the time you received the result, the time you notified the provider, the provider's name, the orders received, and any actions taken. This documentation is your legal record that you fulfilled your obligation. If a patient suffers harm from a critical lab value that was resulted, the investigation will follow a predictable trail: when was the nurse notified, when did the nurse notify the provider, and what happened in between? Gaps in that timeline are where liability lives. Finally, reassess the patient. A critical value is never just a number on a screen — go to the bedside, evaluate the patient for symptoms related to that value, and continue monitoring until the situation stabilizes or new orders are carried out.

Students sometimes feel uncertain about whether it is their place to make these calls, especially early in the program. It is. If you receive a critical result and your instructor is not immediately available, find them urgently or notify the charge nurse. What you never do is wait. Delaying notification of a critical value is one of the most clearly documented causes of preventable patient harm in the literature, and "I wasn't sure if I should call" is not a defense that protects anyone — not the patient, not you, and not your license once you have one.

4.3 Connecting Labs to the Patient in Front of You

Memorizing normal ranges is necessary, but it is not sufficient. The skill that transforms lab knowledge from academic to clinical is the ability to look at your patient's diagnosis and anticipate which lab values are going to matter most before you ever open the chart. When you can do that, you stop being a student who passively reads whatever numbers appear and start becoming a nurse who is actively monitoring for the changes that the disease itself predicts.

Consider the patient admitted with heart failure. Before you look at a single result, you should already be thinking about the labs that tell the story of that disease. BNP — or its variant NT-proBNP — is the biomarker of ventricular stretch, and in heart failure patients, it serves as both a diagnostic and a tracking tool. A BNP that was 900 on admission and has dropped to 340 tells you the diuresis is working and the heart is under less strain. A BNP that continues to rise despite treatment is a red flag. Alongside BNP, you will be watching the BMP closely because the diuretics used to manage fluid overload aggressively pull electrolytes with the water. Potassium, magnesium, and sodium can all shift rapidly in a patient receiving intravenous furosemide, and each of those shifts carries its own set of cardiac risks. BUN and creatinine matter too, because aggressive diuresis can tip a patient into prerenal kidney injury — the provider is trying to dry the patient out enough to relieve the heart without drying them out so much that the kidneys start to fail. You will also check daily weights and strict intake and output, but the labs tell you what the scale cannot: what is happening at the cellular level.

Now consider the diabetic patient. The lab that defines their long-term control is hemoglobin A1c, which reflects average blood glucose over the preceding two to three months. A value below 5.7 percent is considered normal, 5.7 to 6.4 percent indicates prediabetes, and 6.5 percent or above confirms diabetes. A patient with an A1c of 11.2 is telling you, through that single number, that their glucose has been dangerously uncontrolled for months, which reframes everything you are about to do on the clinical floor — their wound healing will be impaired, their infection risk is elevated, and their glucose will be harder to manage during the hospitalization. Day to day, you will be monitoring fingerstick blood glucose before meals and at bedtime, watching for both hyperglycemic spikes and hypoglycemic dips, especially if the patient is receiving insulin on a sliding scale or is NPO for a procedure. The BMP glucose gives you a single-point reading; the A1c gives you the context around it.

The patient on warfarin offers another instructive example. Their PT and INR will be drawn regularly, and you need to know the therapeutic target for their specific indication. A patient with atrial fibrillation is generally managed to an INR of 2.0 to 3.0, while a patient with a mechanical mitral valve may need 2.5 to 3.5. A subtherapeutic INR means the drug is not providing adequate protection against clots. A supratherapeutic INR means bleeding risk is climbing, and the higher it goes, the more urgent the intervention — vitamin K, dose adjustment, or in extreme cases, fresh frozen plasma. You should also know which of your patient's other medications and even dietary habits interact with warfarin, because this is one of the most interaction-prone drugs in the pharmacy and its lab values can swing based on a new antibiotic, a change in diet, or a missed dose.

Patients with renal insufficiency or failure bring yet another lab profile to the foreground. Their BUN and creatinine become daily metrics of kidney function, and the glomerular filtration rate — GFR, often calculated automatically from the creatinine — quantifies how much filtering capacity remains. These values directly impact medication dosing, since drugs cleared by the kidneys accumulate to toxic levels when the kidneys are not keeping up. Electrolyte monitoring is equally critical: potassium climbs when the kidneys cannot excrete it, phosphorus rises, and calcium drops, creating a dangerous metabolic cascade. If the patient is on dialysis, you will be comparing pre- and post-dialysis labs to assess treatment effectiveness.

The pattern across all of these cases is the same. You identify the diagnosis, recall which body systems it threatens, and then focus on the lab values that monitor those systems. Heart failure stresses the heart, kidneys, and electrolytes — so you watch BNP, BMP, and renal function. Diabetes disrupts glucose metabolism — so you watch A1c, fingerstick glucose, and renal markers that track long-term complications. Anticoagulation therapy walks a tightrope between bleeding and clotting — so you watch coagulation studies and hemoglobin. Once you build this habit of diagnosis-driven lab anticipation, you will walk into clinical already knowing which numbers to look for, and your instructor will notice the difference immediately.

This same reasoning connects directly to your next challenge: understanding the medications your patient receives, why they are prescribed, and what you need to assess before you give them. Labs and medications are two halves of the same conversation, and the chapter ahead brings them together.

Chapter 5 — Medication Math and Safe Administration

5.1 The Formulas That Keep Your Patients Safe

Medication errors are among the most common and most preventable causes of patient harm in hospitals, and a significant number of those errors come down to math. Not complicated math — nursing dosage calculations rarely require anything beyond multiplication, division, and the occasional unit conversion — but math performed under pressure, in a busy hallway, with an instructor or a patient waiting. The students who make errors are almost never students who cannot do arithmetic. They are students who do not have a reliable, repeatable method and end up second-guessing themselves halfway through a calculation, switching approaches mid-problem, or skipping the verification step because they feel rushed. This section gives you the formulas you need, walks through them with clinical scenarios you will actually encounter, and establishes a calculation habit that protects your patients and your confidence.

The most versatile formula in nursing math is desired over have, sometimes written as D over H times the vehicle, or quantity on hand. The concept is simple: you know what dose the provider ordered (desired), you know what concentration is available in the medication you are holding (have), and you need to figure out how much to actually administer (the volume or number of tablets). The formula is desired divided by have, multiplied by the vehicle. Suppose a provider orders 250 milligrams of amoxicillin orally, and the pharmacy sends a liquid suspension labeled 125 milligrams per 5 milliliters. Your desired dose is 250 milligrams, your have is 125 milligrams, and the vehicle is 5 milliliters. Divide 250 by 125, which gives you 2, and multiply by 5, which gives you 10 milliliters. That is the volume you draw up and administer. Now consider a scenario with tablets: the order reads metoprolol 75 milligrams by mouth, and the tablets available are scored 25 milligram tablets. Desired is 75, have is 25, vehicle is 1 tablet. 75 divided by 25 equals 3 tablets. Straightforward, but the discipline is in writing it out every time rather than doing it in your head, because the moment you start doing medication math from memory is the moment small mistakes start slipping through.

Weight-based dosing adds one more step, and you will see it frequently in pediatrics, critical care, and with medications like heparin, certain antibiotics, and chemotherapy agents. The order will be written as a dose per kilogram of body weight — for example, 15 milligrams per kilogram per day. Your first job is to ensure you are working in kilograms, not pounds, because mixing up the two is one of the most dangerous errors in weight-based dosing. If the chart lists the patient's weight as 176 pounds, convert by dividing by 2.2 to get 80 kilograms. Then multiply the ordered dose by the weight: 15 milligrams per kilogram times 80 kilograms equals 1,200 milligrams total daily dose. If that dose is divided into three administrations per day, each individual dose is 400 milligrams. From there, use the desired over have formula to determine the volume or number of tablets for each administration. Always double-check your weight conversion before building the rest of the calculation on top of it, because an error at the foundation multiplies through every step above it.

Intravenous drip rate calculations come in two forms, and which one you use depends on whether the IV is running through an electronic infusion pump or a manual gravity setup. For pump-controlled infusions, the provider order or pharmacy label will typically give you a total volume and a time frame — for example, 1,000 milliliters of normal saline to infuse over 8 hours. The formula is total volume in milliliters divided by total time in hours, which gives you milliliters per hour. In this case, 1,000 divided by 8 equals 125 milliliters per hour, and you program the pump accordingly. Where students trip up is when the order gives the time in minutes rather than hours, or when the total volume is something unusual like 250 milliliters over 90 minutes. For the latter, simply divide 250 by 1.5 hours (since 90 minutes is 1.5 hours), which gives approximately 167 milliliters per hour. Always round according to your facility's policy — most pumps accept whole numbers only.

Manual gravity drip rates require one additional piece of information: the drop factor of the tubing, which is printed on the IV tubing package and expressed as drops per milliliter. Standard macrodrip tubing comes in drop factors of 10, 15, or 20 drops per milliliter. Microdrip tubing is always 60 drops per milliliter. The formula is total volume in milliliters divided by total time in minutes, multiplied by the drop factor, which gives you drops per minute. Consider an order for 500 milliliters of lactated Ringer's to infuse over 4 hours using tubing with a drop factor of 15. First convert the time: 4 hours equals 240 minutes. Then calculate: 500 divided by 240 equals approximately 2.08, multiplied by 15 equals approximately 31 drops per minute. You then count the drops in the drip chamber for 15 seconds, multiply by 4, and adjust the roller clamp until you hit your target rate. This skill is less common now that most hospitals use electronic pumps, but you will encounter gravity drips during power outages, in community settings, and on exams, so the formula is worth owning.

There is one more calculation that comes up in clinical practice more often than students anticipate: dosing based on concentration, particularly with high-risk medications. Heparin is a prime example. An order might read "heparin 800 units per hour intravenously," and the bag hanging reads 25,000 units in 500 milliliters of D5W. To find the rate in milliliters per hour, use the desired over have structure adapted for continuous infusions: 800

units per hour divided by the concentration of 25,000 units per 500 milliliters. First, find the concentration per milliliter: 25,000 divided by 500 equals 50 units per milliliter. Then divide the ordered dose by the concentration: 800 divided by 50 equals 16 milliliters per hour. You program the pump to 16, and you label the tubing with the rate, the concentration, and the time you hung the bag. With any high-alert drip — heparin, insulin, dopamine, nitroglycerin — a second nurse will independently verify your calculation before the infusion begins, and that is a safety net you should welcome, not resent.

Across all of these formulas, a few habits make the difference between a student who calculates safely and one who does not. First, always write out the calculation, even when it seems simple enough to do mentally. Written math can be checked; mental math cannot. Second, include your units at every step and cancel them as you go — if the units on your final answer do not match what you expected (milliliters, tablets, drops per minute), something went wrong. Third, apply a reasonableness check before you administer anything. If your calculation tells you to give fifteen tablets of a medication that normally comes as one or two, something is off. If your IV rate comes out to 600 milliliters per hour for a routine antibiotic, recheck it. Common sense is your final safety barrier, and it catches errors that formulas alone cannot. Fourth, when in doubt, ask. No experienced nurse has ever criticized a student for double-checking a dose. The only math mistake that ends a career is the one nobody caught.

5.2 The Six Rights Are Not a Checklist — They Are a Reflex

Every nursing student can recite the six rights of medication administration on command: right patient, right medication, right dose, right route, right time, right documentation. They appear in every pharmacology textbook, on every exam, and in every clinical orientation. And yet medication errors continue to happen in hospitals every single day, not because nurses forgot the list, but because knowing the rights and consistently applying them under real-world conditions are two entirely different things. The distance between recitation and practice is where patients get hurt, and the goal of this section is to turn the six rights from something you memorize into something you physically do, in the same order, every time, until skipping a step feels as wrong as walking out of the house without shoes.

Right patient is first for a reason. Before you open a medication, before you draw up a syringe, before you scan anything, confirm you are standing in front of the correct human being. Use two patient identifiers — full name and date of birth are the standard pair — and verify them against the medication administration record and the patient's wristband. Ask the patient to state their name and birthdate rather than asking "Are you Mrs. Johnson?" because a confused, sedated, or hard-of-hearing patient will sometimes agree with whatever name you suggest. In facilities with barcode scanning, scan the patient's wristband first; the system will reject the medication if there is a mismatch, but only if you actually scan rather than overriding. Students occasionally feel awkward asking a patient they have been caring for all morning to state their name again. Do it anyway. Familiarity is where complacency breeds, and the patient who was in room 204 this morning may have been moved to room 210 while you were at lunch.

Right medication means verifying the drug name, not just glancing at the label. Read the full generic name, because look-alike and sound-alike medications are a well-documented source of error — hydroxyzine and hydralazine, metformin and metronidazole, prednisone and prednisolone. Compare the medication in your hand against the MAR three separate times: when you pull it from the drawer or the automated dispensing cabinet, when you prepare it, and when you are at the bedside ready to give it. Barcode scanning adds a layer of protection, but technology is not infallible; scanners misread damaged barcodes, and overriding alerts becomes dangerously easy once you have done it a few times for legitimate reasons. If the scanner rejects a medication and you cannot identify why, stop and investigate rather than assuming the system is wrong.

Right dose ties directly to the calculations you practiced in the previous section. Confirm that the dose on the MAR matches the dose you have prepared. If the pharmacy sent a different concentration than what you expected, recalculate rather than estimating. If a dose seems unusually high or low for the clinical situation, question it — the order may contain a prescribing error, and catching it is not overstepping, it is exactly what nurses are expected to do. Right route requires verifying whether the medication is oral, intravenous, intramuscular, subcutaneous, topical, rectal, sublingual, or inhaled, because giving a medication by the wrong route can be fatal. An oral medication pushed intravenously or an intramuscular injection given intravenously changes the absorption rate so dramatically that a therapeutic dose can become a lethal one. Right time means administering within the window your facility defines — typically thirty minutes before or after the scheduled time. Some medications are truly time-critical: insulin must align with meals, antibiotics for surgical prophylaxis must be given within the preoperative window, and medications like anticonvulsants and antirejection drugs have narrow therapeutic ranges that cannot tolerate inconsistent timing.

Right documentation closes the loop. Chart the medication, dose, route, time, and your initials immediately after you administer, not before and not two hours later from memory. If the patient refused the medication, document the refusal, the reason if given, and that you notified the provider. An unadministered medication that is not documented as held or refused creates a dangerous gap in the record, because the next nurse may give a double dose assuming the first was missed.

Certain medications carry enough risk that the standard six rights are not sufficient on their own. These are your high-alert medications, and they demand additional safety steps. Insulin requires an independent double-check by a second nurse before administration — both of you verify the type, the dose, the concentration, and the expiration date. Drawing up the wrong type of insulin, particularly confusing rapid-acting with long-acting, is a classic and potentially fatal error. Heparin drips require the same dual verification: two nurses independently confirm the concentration in the bag, the calculated rate, and the pump programming. Intravenous potassium is never given by push — it is always diluted and infused at a controlled rate, typically no faster than 10 milliequivalents per hour on a general floor, because rapid potassium infusion can stop the heart. Opioids require assessment of respiratory rate, sedation level, and pain score before and after administration, with a general hold parameter of a respiratory rate below 12. If any of these high-alert medications make you feel a heightened sense of caution, that feeling is correct, and it should never go away no matter how many years you practice.

5.3 Drug Classes by System — What to Know Before You Give

You will not memorize every medication in the hospital formulary, and you do not need to. What you need is a working knowledge of the major drug classifications organized by body system, so that when you pull a medication you have never seen before, you can identify its class, understand its general mechanism, and know what to assess before and after administration. This section is designed as a rapid reference, not an exhaustive pharmacology review, because what matters at the bedside is whether you can connect the drug to the patient's physiology in the sixty seconds before you walk into the room.

Cardiac medications make up a large portion of what you will administer on a medical-surgical floor. Beta blockers such as metoprolol and atenolol reduce heart rate and blood pressure by blocking the effects of adrenaline on the heart, and your pre-administration assessment is a heart rate and blood pressure — hold for a heart rate below 60 or a systolic below 100 unless the provider has specified different parameters. ACE inhibitors like lisinopril and ARBs like losartan lower blood pressure by disrupting the renin-angiotensin system; watch for a dry cough with ACE inhibitors, which is a known side effect, and monitor potassium because both classes can cause hyperkalemia, especially in patients with renal impairment. Calcium channel blockers such as amlodipine and diltiazem lower blood pressure and, in some cases, slow heart rate; check blood pressure before giving, and be aware that diltiazem and verapamil have more pronounced effects on heart rate than amlodipine. Antiarrhythmics like amiodarone carry serious side effect profiles including thyroid dysfunction, pulmonary toxicity, and liver damage with long-term use, and they require continuous cardiac monitoring during intravenous administration. Diuretics — furosemide being the one you will see most — promote fluid excretion and are a cornerstone of heart failure management; monitor daily weight, intake and output, potassium, and watch for signs of dehydration or electrolyte depletion. Anticoagulants include warfarin, which you monitor with INR, and heparin, which you monitor with aPTT, along with newer direct oral anticoagulants like apixaban and rivarelbaan that require less lab monitoring but carry the same bleeding risks. Before giving any anticoagulant, check the relevant lab value and look for signs of active bleeding.

Respiratory medications center around bronchodilators and corticosteroids. Short-acting beta agonists like albuterol relax bronchial smooth muscle and are used as rescue inhalers; monitor heart rate because tachycardia is a common side effect. Inhaled corticosteroids like fluticasone reduce airway inflammation for maintenance therapy; instruct the patient to rinse their mouth after use to prevent oral candidiasis. Systemic corticosteroids such as prednisone and methylprednisolone suppress inflammation broadly but elevate blood glucose, suppress immune function, and can cause fluid retention — monitor glucose closely in any patient receiving steroids, even those without a diabetes diagnosis.

Endocrine medications in the hospital setting primarily involve insulin and oral hypoglycemics. Rapid-acting insulin such as lispro is given before meals and requires a current blood glucose reading before administration. Long-acting insulin like glargine provides a basal level and is typically given once daily at the same time. Oral agents like metformin lower glucose through different mechanisms and are held before procedures involving contrast dye due to the risk of lactic acidosis. For all glucose-lowering medications, your primary assessment is the blood glucose value, and your primary concern is hypoglycemia — know the symptoms, know where the glucose tablets and D50 are, and never give insulin without checking the number first.

Neurological medications include anticonvulsants, antidepressants, and anxiolytics. Drugs like phenytoin and levetiracetam prevent seizures and often require therapeutic drug level monitoring; phenytoin in particular has a narrow therapeutic range and numerous drug interactions. Benzodiazepines such as lorazepam provide anxiolysis and seizure control but depress respiration, and in elderly patients they significantly increase fall risk. Assess sedation level and respiratory rate before and after administration. Opioid analgesics — morphine, hydromorphone, oxycodone, fentanyl — are used for moderate to severe pain and are the class that demands the most vigilance. Assess pain level, respiratory rate, and sedation score before giving, and reassess within the appropriate timeframe afterward to evaluate effectiveness and watch for respiratory depression. Know that naloxone reverses opioid effects and should be readily accessible whenever opioids are in use.

Gastrointestinal medications include proton pump inhibitors like pantoprazole, which reduce stomach acid production and are commonly given for stress ulcer prophylaxis in hospitalized patients. Antiemetics such as ondansetron control nausea and vomiting; monitor for constipation, which is a frequent side effect. Laxatives and stool softeners — docusate, senna, polyethylene glycol — are used to manage the constipation that hospitalization itself tends to produce, compounded by opioid use and immobility.

The common thread through every class is the same three-part question: what should I check before I give this, what should I watch for while it is working, and what tells me something has gone wrong? Build that habit now, and it will carry you from the first medication you administer as a student through the thousands you will give across your career. With medications covered, the next chapter turns to one of their most common delivery methods — intravenous therapy — and the fluid management principles that accompany it.

Chapter 6 — IV Therapy and Fluid Essentials

6.1 Understanding What Is Running Into Your Patient and Why

Almost every patient you care for during clinical rotations will have some form of intravenous access, and many of them will have fluids running continuously. It becomes so common that students start to tune it out — the IV pole becomes furniture, the bag becomes wallpaper, and the pump becomes background noise. That is a dangerous habit to develop, because what is hanging on that pole and what is delivering it into the patient's bloodstream are clinical decisions with real physiological consequences. Knowing the difference between a peripheral line and a central line, understanding why normal saline was chosen instead of D5W, and being able to explain your patient's fluid therapy during conference are skills that demonstrate you are thinking like a nurse rather than simply performing tasks.

Peripheral intravenous access is the most common type you will encounter and the one you will likely learn to start yourself during nursing school. A peripheral IV is a short catheter — typically 18 to 22 gauge and about an inch to an inch and a quarter long — inserted into a superficial vein, usually in the forearm or hand. It is appropriate for short-term therapy, typically 72 to 96 hours before the site should be evaluated for rotation, and it can handle most standard infusions: hydration fluids, antibiotics, pain medications, and blood products through an appropriately large-gauge catheter. The limitations of a peripheral line are reach and durability. Because the catheter sits in a small, superficial vein, it cannot tolerate highly concentrated solutions, caustic medications like vasopressors, or prolonged total parenteral nutrition, all of which would damage the vessel wall. Site assessment is your responsibility on every shift: inspect for redness, swelling, warmth, tenderness, and any leakage around the insertion point. If the patient reports pain at the site or you notice any of those signs, the line needs to come out — continuing to infuse through a compromised peripheral IV risks infiltration, where fluid leaks into surrounding tissue, or phlebitis, where the vein itself becomes inflamed. Both are preventable if you are paying attention.

Midline catheters occupy a middle ground that students often overlook. A midline is longer than a peripheral IV — usually about eight inches — and is inserted into a vein in the upper arm, typically the basilic or cephalic vein, but the tip does not advance into central vasculature. It stays in the peripheral venous system, just in a larger and more stable vessel. Midlines are chosen when the patient needs IV access for one to four weeks but does not require a central line. They can handle most antibiotics, hydration fluids, and some medications that would irritate a shorter peripheral catheter, but they are still not appropriate for vesicant drugs, TPN, or solutions with extreme pH or osmolality. Nursing care for a midline includes regular dressing changes, site assessment, and monitoring arm circumference for signs of deep vein thrombosis, which is a known complication.

Peripherally inserted central catheters — PICCs — are where the conversation shifts to central access. A PICC is inserted into a peripheral vein in the upper arm, but the catheter is long enough to thread all the way through to the superior vena cava, making it a central line despite its peripheral insertion point. PICCs are used for patients who need weeks to months of IV therapy: long-term antibiotics, chemotherapy, TPN, or frequent blood draws. They can have single, double, or triple lumens, allowing multiple incompatible infusions to run simultaneously. Nursing students are generally allowed to assess PICC sites, perform dressing changes with proper sterile technique once checked off on the skill, flush lumens, and administer medications through them under supervision. What you are typically not permitted to do is insert or remove a PICC — that is performed by a specially trained nurse or interventional radiology. Site care follows strict sterile protocol: a transparent semipermeable dressing that allows visual inspection, changed every seven days or when soiled, with chlorhexidine antisepsis and careful stabilization to prevent migration. Measure and document the external catheter length at every dressing change, because a PICC that has migrated may no longer have its tip in the proper position, which changes what can safely be infused through it.

Non-tunneled central venous catheters are inserted directly into large central veins — the internal jugular, subclavian, or femoral — with the tip resting in the superior vena cava or at the junction of the superior vena cava and the right atrium. These are typically placed by physicians or advanced practice providers at the bedside or in a procedure suite, and they are used in acute and critical care settings for hemodynamic monitoring, rapid volume resuscitation, vasopressor administration, and situations where peripheral access is impossible. Tunneled catheters and implanted ports are variations designed for long-term or permanent access, commonly seen in oncology patients or those requiring chronic therapies like dialysis. As a student, your role with central venous catheters is assessment and maintenance under supervision — monitoring the site for infection, performing sterile dressing changes, flushing lumens, and understanding which lumen is designated for which purpose in a multi-lumen catheter. Central line-associated bloodstream infections are a significant and measurable patient safety metric, and meticulous aseptic technique during every interaction with a central line is not optional, it is the standard of care.

With access understood, turn your attention to what is actually in the bag. Intravenous fluids are categorized by their tonicity relative to blood plasma, and that single characteristic determines how the fluid behaves once it enters the bloodstream. Isotonic solutions have the same osmolality as plasma — roughly 270 to 310 milliosmoles per liter — which means they stay in the intravascular space without causing fluid to shift into or out of cells. Normal saline, which is 0.9 percent sodium chloride, is the workhorse isotonic fluid and is used for volume resuscitation, dehydration, blood product administration, and as a compatible carrier for most IV medications. Lactated Ringer's is another isotonic solution that includes electrolytes — sodium, potassium, calcium, and lactate — and is commonly used in surgical patients, trauma resuscitation, and burn care. The key consideration with normal saline in large volumes is the risk of hyperchloremic metabolic acidosis, because you are infusing a significant chloride load; lactated Ringer's avoids that issue but is incompatible with certain medications and with blood products in the same line because the calcium can cause clotting.

Hypotonic solutions have a lower osmolality than plasma, which means water shifts out of the vascular space and into the cells. Half-normal saline, or 0.45 percent sodium chloride, is the most common hypotonic fluid, and it is typically used for patients who need free water replacement — those with hypernatremia or cellular dehydration. The danger of hypotonic fluids is giving too much, because excess water shifting into cells can cause cellular swelling, and in the brain, that swelling becomes cerebral edema. Hypotonic fluids are generally infused slowly and are contraindicated in patients with increased intracranial pressure, burns, or liver disease with third-spacing.

Hypertonic solutions have a higher osmolality than plasma, pulling water out of cells and into the vascular space. Three percent saline is the classic hypertonic fluid, reserved for severe symptomatic hyponatremia — seizures, altered mental status — where rapid correction of sodium is necessary. It is administered in a monitored setting, often the ICU, with frequent sodium level checks because correcting too quickly carries the risk of osmotic demyelination syndrome, a devastating neurological complication. D10W and D50W — dextrose solutions at 10 and 50 percent — are hypertonic and used for hypoglycemia management. TPN solutions are also hypertonic and must be infused through central access because their high osmolality would destroy peripheral veins.

When your instructor asks during conference why your patient is on lactated Ringer's at 125 milliliters per hour instead of normal saline, they are not asking you to recite a textbook definition. They are asking whether you understand that this post-operative patient needs volume and electrolyte replacement without the chloride load that liters of normal saline would bring. That is the level of understanding that separates a student who is managing tasks from a student who is managing a patient, and it is entirely within your reach once you start looking at the IV pole as a clinical decision rather than a piece of equipment.

6.2 When the Pump Alarms — Flow Rates, Programming, and Troubleshooting

You already learned the core IV rate formulas in Chapter 5, so this section focuses on what happens after the math — the practical reality of programming a pump, managing an infusion, and responding when something goes wrong. Because something will go wrong. IV pumps alarm constantly, and the student who stands frozen staring at a beeping machine while the patient watches nervously is a student who has not been taught what the alarms mean or what to do about them. By the end of this section, you will know.

Start with the pump itself. Most facilities use smart infusion pumps that include drug libraries — pre-programmed dose limits designed to prevent catastrophic errors. When you program an infusion, you will typically select the drug or fluid from the library, enter the ordered rate in milliliters per hour, and confirm the volume to be infused. The pump then monitors the infusion and alerts you when the bag is nearly empty, when it detects an occlusion, or when it senses air in the line. Pay attention to the volume-to-be-infused setting, because this is what tells the pump when to stop. If you forget to set it, the pump will continue until the bag runs dry and air enters the tubing. When you hang a new bag, always verify three things before pressing start: the rate matches the order, the correct channel is selected if the pump has multiple channels, and the tubing is loaded properly through the pumping mechanism. A tubing segment that is not seated correctly will either alarm immediately or deliver an inaccurate rate, both of which waste time and erode your patient's confidence in you.

Now for the complications, because recognizing them early is the single most important IV management skill you can develop. Infiltration occurs when the catheter tip dislodges from the vein or punctures through the vessel wall, allowing fluid to leak into the surrounding subcutaneous tissue. The classic signs are swelling at or above the insertion site, skin that feels cool to the touch compared to the surrounding area, pallor, and the patient reporting tightness or discomfort. The infusion may slow down or the pump may alarm with an occlusion message because the fluid is meeting increased resistance as it pools in tissue rather than flowing through the vein. When you identify an infiltration, stop the infusion immediately, disconnect the tubing, remove the catheter, and elevate the affected extremity to encourage reabsorption of the fluid. Document the event, including the appearance of the site and the approximate amount of swelling, and notify the provider if a vesicant medication was infusing, because vesicant infiltration — called extravasation — causes tissue necrosis and requires specific antidotes and interventions depending on the drug involved.

Phlebitis is inflammation of the vein, and it presents differently than infiltration. The hallmark signs are redness streaking along the course of the vein, warmth at and above the insertion site, tenderness that the patient reports even without palpation, and sometimes a palpable hardened cord where the vein has become inflamed. Phlebitis can be mechanical, caused by the catheter irritating the vessel wall; chemical, caused by the pH or osmolality of the medication or fluid; or infectious, caused by bacterial contamination. Regardless of the cause, the intervention is the same in the acute setting: discontinue the infusion, remove the catheter, apply a warm compress to the affected area, and start a new IV in a different location, preferably in the opposite extremity. If you suspect infectious phlebitis — particularly if there is purulent drainage at the insertion site or the patient has developed a fever — notify the provider, because the catheter tip may need to be cultured.

Occlusion alarms are the most common pump alarm you will hear, and they can result from multiple causes. A kinked or clamped line is the simplest fix — trace the tubing from the pump to the patient and look for bends, pinches, or a closed clamp that was left shut after a previous disconnection. If the tubing is clear, check whether the patient is lying on the line or has bent their arm in a way that compresses the catheter. Positional occlusions resolve when the patient straightens the limb or shifts their weight. If neither of those interventions clears the alarm, the catheter itself may be occluded — a fibrin sheath or small clot at the tip can block flow, and attempting to force the flush risks pushing the clot into the bloodstream. Notify your instructor or the assigned nurse, as occluded central lines sometimes require a thrombolytic flush ordered by the provider.

Air in the tubing causes alarm in both senses of the word — the pump detects it and the student panics. In reality, small air bubbles in peripheral IV tubing are common and rarely dangerous; the volume of air needed to cause a clinically significant air embolism in an adult is estimated at several milliliters per kilogram, far more than the tiny bubbles you see traveling through the line. That said, you should still remove them, because best practice is best practice and patients who see bubbles heading toward their arm become understandably frightened. To clear air from the line, pause the infusion, use the pump's air-removal function if available, or disconnect the tubing at a port below the air, let the fluid push the air out, and reconnect. For large amounts of air, re-prime the line entirely. If you suspect a significant air embolism — sudden dyspnea, chest pain, hypotension, altered mental status — place the patient on their left side in Trendelenburg position to trap the air in the right atrium and call for help immediately.

6.3 Blood Products, Electrolyte Replacement, and the High-Stakes Side of Fluid Management

Blood product administration is one of the most protocol-heavy skills in nursing, and for good reason: a transfusion reaction can kill a patient within minutes, and the errors that cause the worst reactions are almost always human ones — wrong blood hung on the wrong patient. The safety system exists to make that mistake nearly impossible, but only if every step is followed without shortcuts.

The process begins before the blood ever arrives on the unit. The provider orders the transfusion, and the lab performs a type and crossmatch, testing the patient's blood against donor units to confirm compatibility. When the blood product arrives — whether it is packed red blood cells, fresh frozen plasma, platelets, or cryoprecipitate — two qualified staff members must verify it at the bedside. Both nurses independently check the patient's identity against their wristband, compare the blood bank tag on the unit to the patient's blood bank bracelet, verify the unit number on the bag matches the compatibility report, confirm the blood type and Rh factor, inspect the bag for discoloration or clots, and check the expiration date. Every one of those checks must match perfectly. A single discrepancy means the product does not get hung until the issue is resolved, period. No exceptions, no matter how busy the floor is.

Once verified, the blood product is infused through a dedicated blood administration set with an in-line filter, using normal saline as the only compatible flush — never lactated Ringer's, never dextrose, as both can damage the blood cells or cause clotting in the line. The infusion begins slowly, typically at about two milliliters per minute for the first fifteen minutes, because the majority of severe transfusion reactions declare themselves early. During those first fifteen minutes, you stay with the patient. Take a full set of vital signs before starting, then again at fifteen minutes, and monitor for the signs of a transfusion reaction: fever, chills, rigors, flank or back pain, chest tightness, dyspnea, hives or flushing, hypotension, tachycardia, or a sense of impending doom that the patient may describe as something just feeling terribly wrong. If any of those signs appear, stop the transfusion immediately, keep the IV line open with normal saline, stay with the patient, and call for help. The blood bag and tubing are saved and sent back to the blood bank for investigation. Vital signs are taken again, and the provider is notified for further orders, which may include antihistamines, antipyretics, epinephrine, or in the case of a hemolytic reaction, aggressive fluid resuscitation and close monitoring for renal failure. After the first fifteen minutes, if the patient is tolerating the transfusion, vital signs are repeated at intervals per your facility policy — commonly every thirty minutes and at completion — and the unit is typically infused within two to four hours, as blood left at room temperature beyond four hours must be discarded due to bacterial growth risk.

Electrolyte replacement by the intravenous route is the other high-vigilance fluid scenario you will encounter regularly. Potassium replacement is the most common and the most dangerous. Intravenous potassium chloride is always diluted and never given by push — this is a rule that admits no exception, because a rapid bolus of potassium can cause fatal cardiac arrest. On a general medical-surgical floor, the typical maximum infusion rate is 10 milliequivalents per hour through a peripheral line, and higher rates require cardiac monitoring and central access. The infusion often burns, and patients will tell you the IV site hurts — slowing the rate, applying a warm pack over the site, and ensuring adequate dilution all help, but some discomfort is expected. Monitor the patient's cardiac rhythm if they are on telemetry, and recheck the potassium level after replacement to confirm the deficit has been corrected.

Magnesium replacement follows a similar framework. Intravenous magnesium sulfate is infused slowly, typically one to two grams over one to two hours, and rapid infusion can cause flushing, hypotension, and respiratory depression. Monitor blood pressure and respiratory rate during the infusion, and be aware that magnesium toxicity depresses deep tendon reflexes — checking patellar reflexes is a classic bedside assessment during magnesium administration, particularly in obstetric patients receiving it for preeclampsia.

Calcium replacement is less common on general floors but critical when it occurs. Calcium gluconate is preferred over calcium chloride for peripheral infusions because calcium chloride is highly caustic and can destroy a peripheral vein. Infuse calcium slowly with cardiac monitoring, since rapid administration can cause bradycardia and cardiac arrest. Never infuse calcium and phosphorus through the same line or simultaneously, as they will precipitate and form crystite particles that can embolize.

Across all of these high-stakes infusions, the pattern is the same: verify the order, verify the product, verify the rate, monitor the patient closely during administration, and know exactly what a complication looks like so you can act before it escalates. These skills bridge directly into the hands-on clinical procedures covered in the next chapter, where the tools in your hands demand the same combination of knowledge, technique, and vigilance.

Chapter 7 — Essential Clinical Procedures

7.1 The Skills Your Hands Need to Know

There is a difference between understanding a procedure conceptually and standing at the bedside with a sterile field open and a patient watching you. The gap between those two realities is where most student anxiety lives, and it does not close by reading more — it closes by having a clear, reliable sequence in your head before you glove up. This section walks through the procedures nursing students perform most frequently during clinical rotations, not as a replacement for your skills lab practice, but as a quick-access reference you can review in the hallway sixty seconds before you walk into the room. Know the indication, gather the supplies, follow the steps in order, and assess afterward. That framework applies to every procedure in nursing, and these four are where you will use it first.

Foley catheter insertion is often the first invasive procedure students perform on a real patient, and the stakes feel enormous in the moment even though the skill itself is straightforward once you have the sequence down. A Foley — an indwelling urinary catheter — is indicated when accurate urine output monitoring is essential, when the patient has acute urinary retention, during certain surgical procedures, for bladder irrigation, or in select cases of immobility where skin integrity is at serious risk from incontinence. Before you open anything, confirm the order, verify the patient's identity, explain the procedure and what the patient will feel, ensure privacy, and position the patient appropriately — supine with knees bent and apart for female patients, supine with legs slightly apart for male patients. Perform hand hygiene and set up your sterile field using the contents of the catheter insertion kit, which typically includes the catheter itself, a prefilled syringe for balloon inflation, sterile gloves, drapes, antiseptic solution, lubricant, a specimen cup, and a collection bag. The critical principle through the entire procedure is sterile technique: once your dominant hand is gloved and designated as your sterile hand, it touches only sterile supplies and the catheter itself. Your non-dominant hand becomes your non-sterile hand and handles the patient's anatomy. If at any point you suspect contamination — the catheter tip touches the bed linens, your sterile glove brushes the patient's thigh, anything — stop and get a new kit. A urinary tract infection caused by a contaminated insertion is a preventable harm, and starting over costs five minutes while an infection costs the patient days.

For female patients, use your non-dominant hand to separate the labia and identify the urethral meatus, which sits between the clitoris and the vaginal opening. Cleanse with antiseptic swabs, working from front to back, using a fresh swab for each stroke, and do not let the labia close once you have prepped the area. With your sterile hand, pick up the lubricated catheter and insert gently until urine flows, then advance another inch or two to ensure the balloon is well within the bladder before inflating. For male patients, hold the penis at a 90-degree angle to the body with your non-dominant hand, retract the foreskin if present, cleanse the meatus in circular motions moving outward, and insert the well-lubricated catheter slowly and steadily. You may meet slight resistance at the level of the prostate — maintain gentle, consistent pressure and ask the patient to take deep breaths, which relaxes the external sphincter. Never force the catheter. Once urine flows, advance a few more inches before inflating the balloon with the prefilled syringe. If the patient reports sharp pain during inflation, deflate immediately, advance further, and try again, because the balloon may be sitting in the urethra rather than the bladder. Secure the catheter to the patient's thigh with the provided securement device to prevent traction on the urethra, ensure the drainage bag hangs below the level of the bladder but never touches the floor, and document the procedure including catheter size, balloon volume, urine characteristics, and the patient's tolerance.

Nasogastric tube insertion is uncomfortable for the patient and nerve-racking for the student, but it follows a logical sequence that becomes manageable with practice. An NG tube is indicated for gastric decompression — removing air and fluid from the stomach to relieve distension, nausea, or obstruction — or for enteral feeding or medication delivery when the patient cannot swallow safely. Gather your supplies: the appropriate-size NG tube, water-soluble lubricant, a syringe for aspiration, pH testing strips, tape or a bridle securement device, a suction canister or feeding pump depending on the purpose, and a cup of water with a straw if the patient is allowed to swallow. Measure the tube before insertion by placing the tip at the patient's nose, extending to the earlobe, and then down to the xiphoid process; mark that distance on the tube, because it estimates the length needed to reach the stomach. Position the patient sitting upright with the head slightly flexed forward — not extended backward, which opens the airway instead of the esophagus. Lubricate the tip of the tube generously and insert into the nostril, directing it straight back along the floor of the nasal passage, not upward. When the tube reaches the posterior pharynx, the patient will feel the urge to gag, and this is where coaching matters: ask them to take small sips of water through the straw and swallow as you continue advancing. The swallowing closes the epiglottis over the trachea and helps guide the tube into the esophagus rather than the airway. If the patient begins coughing violently, becomes cyanotic, or cannot speak, the tube may have entered the trachea — withdraw it immediately and allow the patient to recover before reattempting. Once the tube is advanced to your measured mark, confirm placement. The gold standard is a chest X-ray, but at the bedside, aspirate gastric contents and test the pH — a reading of 5.5 or below suggests gastric placement. Auscultation alone, the old practice of injecting air and listening for a whoosh over the stomach, is no longer considered reliable for confirming placement. Secure the tube to the nose with tape or a commercial device, connect it to low intermittent suction or a feeding system as ordered, and document the insertion including the centimeter mark at the nostril, the method of placement verification, the character of any aspirate, and the patient's response.

Wound care and dressing changes are procedures you will perform across virtually every clinical specialty, and the principles remain constant even though wound types vary enormously. Before you begin, review the wound care order to understand what cleansing solution to use, what type of dressing to apply, and whether any topical medications or packing are indicated. Gather all supplies before opening anything so you are not leaving a patient with an exposed wound while you search for another pack of gauze. Remove the old dressing carefully, noting the type, amount, color, and odor of any drainage on the old dressing itself — this is assessment data, not trash. Observe the wound bed: healthy granulation tissue appears beefy red, slough is yellow and stringy, and eschar is black, hard, and leathery. Measure the wound's length, width, and depth if your facility requires it, and note the condition of the surrounding skin — maceration from excessive moisture, erythema from spreading infection, or undermining and tunneling that indicate the wound extends beneath intact skin edges. Cleanse the wound as ordered, typically with normal saline using gentle irrigation rather than scrubbing, working from the cleanest area to the least clean. Apply the prescribed dressing using clean or sterile technique as the wound type dictates — surgical incisions generally require sterile technique, while chronic wounds managed with moist wound healing may use clean technique per facility protocol. Secure the dressing, label it with the date, time, and your initials, and document everything you observed, including your comparison to the last documented wound assessment.

Ostomy care rounds out the procedures you are most likely to encounter as a student. A patient with an ostomy — colostomy, ileostomy, or urostomy — requires regular pouching system changes, and while a wound-ostomy nurse specialist handles complex issues, the routine care falls to the bedside nurse. Assess the stoma each time you change the appliance: it should be pink to red, moist, and slightly raised above the skin surface. A stoma that appears dusky, dark, or pale may have compromised blood flow and needs to be reported. Gently remove the existing pouching system, cleanse the peristomal skin with warm water — no soap or adhesive removers unless specifically approved, as residue interferes with the next seal — and pat dry thoroughly. Measure the stoma or use a pre-cut wafer that fits snugly around it, leaving no more than an eighth of an inch of exposed skin between the stoma and the wafer edge, because exposed skin will break down from effluent contact. Apply stoma paste or barrier rings if needed to fill uneven skin contours, press the wafer firmly in place, and attach the pouch. Empty the pouch when it is one-third to one-half full, because a heavy pouch pulls on the seal and causes leaks. Document stoma appearance, output characteristics, peristomal skin condition, and the patient's participation in care, since teaching the patient to manage their own ostomy is a central nursing goal from the day of surgery forward.

Each of these procedures will feel clumsy the first time, better the second, and almost natural by the fourth or fifth. The sequence is always the same: know why you are doing it, have everything ready, maintain your technique, and assess the result. Review these steps in the hallway before you walk in, and you will find that your hands remember far more than you expected.

7.2 Collecting Specimens Without Contaminating Them, and Delivering Oxygen Without Guessing

Specimen collection sounds simple until you get the results back and the lab reports that the sample was contaminated, improperly collected, or insufficient in volume, and suddenly the provider is ordering a repeat, the patient is annoyed, and your instructor is asking what went wrong. The techniques themselves are not difficult, but the margin between a usable specimen and a useless one is often a single misstep — a forgotten cleansing wipe, a container that touched the toilet bowl rim, a swab that grazed intact skin before entering the wound bed. Master the details now and you will save yourself and your patients a significant amount of frustration.

Blood glucose monitoring is the specimen procedure you will perform most often, sometimes multiple times per shift on a single patient. The process is quick but demands attention to accuracy. Begin by confirming the order and checking whether the reading is due before a meal, after a meal, at bedtime, or at a specific time related to an insulin protocol. Verify that the glucometer has been quality-controlled per your facility's schedule and that the test strips are not expired, because expired strips produce unreliable numbers. Perform hand hygiene and glove up. The preferred site is the side of the fingertip rather than the pad, where there are fewer nerve endings and blood flow is still adequate. Wipe the site with alcohol and allow it to dry completely — residual alcohol dilutes the blood drop and can falsely lower the result. Use the lancet device to puncture the skin, wipe away the first drop of blood with clean gauze, and apply the second drop to the test strip, because the first drop contains interstitial fluid that can skew the reading. Once the meter displays the result, document it, compare it to the patient's sliding scale or insulin order, and take the appropriate action. If the result seems inconsistent with the patient's clinical presentation — a reading of 42 in a patient who is sitting up chatting and eating crackers, for instance — recheck before treating, because technical errors do happen.

Urine specimen collection varies depending on the test ordered. A clean-catch midstream specimen is the most common and is used for urinalysis and culture. The patient cleanses the periurethral area with the provided antiseptic wipes — front to back in female patients, cleaning the urethral meatus in male patients — begins voiding into the toilet, then catches the midstream portion in the sterile cup without stopping the flow. The first part of the stream flushes bacteria from the distal urethra, and the midstream portion reflects what is actually in the bladder. The most frequent contamination error is failing to cleanse adequately or allowing the cup to touch the inner thigh or toilet, introducing skin flora that the lab then reports as a false positive infection. For patients with an indwelling catheter, specimens are drawn from the sampling port on the catheter tubing using aseptic technique after clamping the tubing below the port for fifteen to thirty minutes to allow fresh urine to accumulate — never disconnect the drainage bag and pour from it, because that urine has been sitting at room temperature and is bacterially unreliable. Twenty-four-hour urine collections test for substances like creatinine clearance, protein, or cortisol that require a full day's output. The process begins by having the patient void and discarding that first specimen to establish the start time, then collecting every subsequent void in the provided container, which is typically kept on ice or refrigerated, for exactly twenty-four hours, including the final void at the end of the collection period. A single missed void invalidates the entire test, so patient education about the importance of catching every drop is essential.

Wound cultures require a technique that many students get wrong on the first attempt. The goal is to sample the organisms actually infecting the wound, not the surface bacteria that colonize every open wound to some degree. Cleanse the wound first with normal saline to remove surface debris and contaminants. Then use the culture swab in the area of the wound bed that appears most actively infected — the reddest, most exudative tissue — pressing firmly enough to express fluid from the tissue and rotating the swab as you move it across a one-centimeter-square area using a zigzag pattern for about five seconds. Swabbing only the surface or the wound edges catches colonizing bacteria rather than the causative pathogen and leads to misleading culture results. Place the swab in the transport medium, label it, and send it to the lab promptly. Stool specimens follow facility-specific protocols depending on the test — a standard stool culture, Clostridioides difficile testing, or occult blood screening each have different collection requirements. For C. difficile, the stool must be liquid or unformed, as the lab will reject formed stool. For occult blood testing, remind the patient about dietary restrictions that can cause false positives, such as red meat and certain vegetables, and ensure the specimen is collected per the specific card or container instructions provided.

Oxygen delivery is the other domain where students frequently hesitate because they are unsure which device matches the patient's needs and what flow rate to set. A nasal cannula is the first-line device for mild to moderate hypoxemia, delivering roughly 24 to 44 percent oxygen at flow rates of one to six liters per minute. It is comfortable, allows the patient to eat and talk, and is appropriate for most floor patients who need supplemental oxygen. Above six liters, a nasal cannula dries the nasal mucosa excessively and provides diminishing returns in oxygen concentration, so you transition to a mask. A simple face mask delivers 40 to 60 percent oxygen at five to ten liters per minute — the minimum flow must be at least five liters to prevent rebreathing of exhaled carbon dioxide that accumulates inside the mask. A non-rebreather mask is reserved for acute hypoxemia requiring high-concentration oxygen, delivering up to 90 to 100 percent at ten to fifteen liters per minute; the reservoir bag must remain at least two-thirds inflated during inspiration, and if it collapses, the flow rate is insufficient. High-flow nasal cannula systems deliver heated, humidified oxygen at precisely controlled concentrations and flow rates up to 60 liters per minute, and they are increasingly used in step-down and ICU settings for patients with severe respiratory failure who might otherwise require intubation. When adjusting any oxygen device, always correlate the flow rate with the patient's oxygen saturation, respiratory effort, and level of consciousness, and remember that in patients with chronic carbon dioxide retention — predominantly those with advanced COPD — excessive oxygen can blunt the hypoxic respiratory drive, so target saturations are typically set lower, around 88 to 92 percent, per the provider's order.

7.3 Managing Tubes and Drains Without Losing Your Nerve

Patients returning from surgery frequently arrive with one or more drainage devices in place, and the sight of fluid-filled tubing emerging from a patient's body can be unsettling the first time you encounter it. The discomfort passes quickly once you understand what each device does, what the output should look like, and what constitutes a problem. Your job with any drain is consistent: assess, measure, document, and maintain patency — and know when to call for help.

Chest tubes are the most intimidating drain students encounter, largely because the stakes are visibly high. A chest tube is placed into the pleural space to evacuate air, blood, or fluid that is preventing the lung from fully expanding. The tube connects to a closed drainage system — most commonly a compact three-chamber unit that combines a collection chamber, a water seal chamber, and a suction control chamber in a single disposable device. Your assessment begins with the patient: are they breathing comfortably, is their oxygen saturation stable, and do they report worsening dyspnea or chest pain? Then assess the system. The water seal chamber should show gentle tidaling — the water level rising and falling with the patient's respirations — which confirms the system is communicating with the pleural space. Continuous vigorous bubbling in the water seal chamber suggests an air leak, which could be at the insertion site, at a tubing connection, or in the lung itself. Check all connections for tightness, inspect the dressing, and if the bubbling persists, notify the provider. The collection chamber receives the drainage, and you should mark the fluid level with the time at the start of every shift and monitor output hourly in the early postoperative period. Drainage that is initially bloody should gradually transition to serosanguineous — a light pink, watery appearance. A sudden increase in output, particularly more than 200 milliliters in a single hour of bright red blood, is an emergency that demands immediate provider notification. Never raise the drainage system above the level of the patient's chest, as this can allow fluid to flow back into the pleural space, and never clamp a chest tube without a specific provider order, because clamping in the presence of an air leak can rapidly produce a tension pneumothorax.

Jackson-Pratt drains and Hemovac drains are closed-suction devices used to remove fluid from surgical sites and prevent hematoma or seroma formation. A Jackson-Pratt consists of a flexible, perforated tube connected to a grenade-shaped bulb that creates gentle suction when compressed. A Hemovac operates on the same principle but uses a flat, disk-shaped reservoir that generates higher suction. For both devices, your assessment includes inspecting the insertion site for signs of infection, checking that the drain is secured to the patient's skin or gown to prevent accidental dislodgement, and emptying the collection reservoir when it is half full or at scheduled intervals. To empty, remove the plug, pour the contents into a graduated measuring container, squeeze the reservoir flat to reestablish suction, replace the plug while maintaining compression, and document the volume, color, and consistency of the output. Normal drainage evolves from sanguineous in the immediate postoperative period to serosanguineous over the following days. Output that suddenly increases, becomes frankly bloody after it had begun clearing, develops a foul odor, or becomes purulent should be reported. Patients sometimes become alarmed by the appearance of the fluid, so take a moment to explain what they are seeing and reassure them that the drain is doing exactly what it is supposed to do.

Other surgical drains you may encounter include Penrose drains, which are open drains that rely on gravity rather than suction and require absorbent dressings over the exit site that you will change as they become saturated. Because they are open systems, infection risk is higher, and meticulous site care matters. Blake drains function similarly to Jackson-Pratt drains but use a channeled design that allows drainage even when tissue collapses around the tube, making them common in thoracic and abdominal surgeries.

When mobilizing any patient with a tube or drain, the priority is preventing dislodgement. Secure the drainage system to the patient's gown below the insertion site so that standing, turning, or walking does not create traction. Walk on the side of the drain so you can monitor it, and teach the patient to hold the collection device below their waist when ambulating. For patients with chest tubes, the drainage unit has a handle or hook — carry it upright and below chest level, and never let tubing loop on the floor where a foot could catch it. Before any position change, trace each line from the patient outward to confirm nothing will be pulled, caught, or kinked. The few seconds that check takes can prevent a painful and potentially dangerous accidental removal.

All output from every drain must be documented with the same specificity you bring to any clinical finding: volume in milliliters, color, consistency, odor if present, and the time frame of the measurement. These numbers become the trend that tells the surgical team whether the patient is healing normally or developing a complication, and incomplete documentation erases that trend. The charting and documentation practices you will need for this and every other clinical task are covered in full in the chapter ahead.

Chapter 8 — Charting and Clinical Documentation

8.1 Four Frameworks, One Goal: A Note That Protects Your Patient and Your License

Documentation is the part of nursing that nobody enters the profession to do, and yet it may be the single most consequential skill you develop. What you chart becomes the legal record of what happened to the patient during your care. If it was not documented, the legal standard holds that it was not done — not assessed, not communicated, not administered, not observed. That principle sounds like a cliché until you are sitting in a deposition three years from now and the only evidence of what you did or did not do on a particular shift is the note you wrote. Every entry you make should be written with the understanding that a stranger — a lawyer, a judge, a jury member with no medical background — may one day read it and use it to reconstruct what happened. That is not meant to frighten you. It is meant to make you take charting as seriously as you take the assessment itself, because in the eyes of the law, the chart is the assessment.

Before you can write well, you need to understand the framework your facility uses, because hospitals and nursing programs do not all document the same way. The four most common structures you will encounter are SBAR, DAR, SOAP, and narrative notes. Each one organizes clinical information differently, but all of them share the same underlying purpose: capturing what you found, what it means, and what you did about it in a format that another clinician can quickly read and act on.

SBAR stands for Situation, Background, Assessment, and Recommendation, and while it is most commonly associated with verbal handoff communication and phone calls to providers, many facilities also use it as a written documentation format for shift notes and event reporting. The Situation is a concise statement of what is happening right now — the patient's name, room number, and the immediate reason you are writing. The Background provides the clinical context: admitting diagnosis, relevant medical history, current medications, recent procedures, and any changes from baseline. The Assessment is your clinical interpretation of the situation — not just the raw data, but what you believe it means based on your nursing judgment. And the Recommendation is what you are suggesting, requesting, or planning to do next. A written SBAR note for a patient whose blood pressure dropped might read: Situation — patient in room 312 experienced a systolic blood pressure drop from 132 to 88 over the past two hours. Background — the patient is a 67-year-old male, postoperative day one following right hip arthroplasty, with a history of hypertension managed with lisinopril, which was administered at 0800 this morning; hemoglobin this morning was 9.2, down from 11.4 preoperatively. Assessment — the blood pressure trend in the context of declining hemoglobin raises concern for postoperative bleeding; the patient reports lightheadedness when sitting up and appears pale. Recommendation — requested provider evaluation, recommended a stat hemoglobin and hematocrit, and held the next scheduled antihypertensive pending reassessment. That note tells the complete story in a structured, scannable format that any clinician picking up the chart can follow instantly.

DAR stands for Data, Action, and Response, and it is the framework used in focus charting, a system where each note is organized around a specific patient focus — a nursing diagnosis, a sign or symptom, a change in condition, or an event. The Data section captures subjective and objective findings related to that focus. The Action section records what you did about it —

interventions, treatments, notifications, education. The Response section documents how the patient responded to your interventions. A DAR note focused on pain management might read: Focus — acute pain. Data — patient rates pain at 8 out of 10 in the right lower abdomen, described as sharp and constant, grimacing with movement, guarding on palpation, last analgesic administered four hours ago. Action — administered hydromorphone 0.5 milligrams intravenously per order at 1420, repositioned patient to left side with pillow support, dimmed room lighting, assessed for potential surgical complications contributing to pain. Response — at 1450 patient reports pain at 4 out of 10, facial expression relaxed, able to take deep breaths without grimacing, resting comfortably. That single entry captures the clinical story of one problem from identification through intervention to outcome, and a series of these entries across a shift builds a comprehensive picture of the patient's day.

SOAP notes — Subjective, Objective, Assessment, and Plan — are the framework most associated with provider documentation, but many nursing programs teach them and some facilities use them for nursing notes as well. The Subjective section records what the patient tells you in their own words: symptoms, complaints, concerns, and their description of how they feel. The Objective section captures your measurable, observable findings: vital signs, physical examination results, lab values, intake and output, wound measurements, and any other data you can quantify or directly observe. The Assessment section is your clinical interpretation — what the combined subjective and objective data suggest about the patient's status. The Plan describes the actions to be taken: continuing current interventions, adjusting medications, scheduling follow-up tests, consulting other services, or modifying the care plan. A SOAP note for a patient with worsening respiratory status might read: Subjective — patient states "I feel like I can't get a deep breath, it started about an hour ago and it's getting worse." Objective — respiratory rate 26, oxygen saturation 89 percent on two liters nasal cannula, bilateral crackles noted in lower lung fields, previously clear at 0700 assessment, heart rate 108, blood pressure 142/88, no fever, BNP pending. Assessment — new onset of dyspnea with bilateral crackles and tachycardia suggests possible fluid overload versus hospital-acquired pneumonia; clinical picture is consistent with worsening heart failure exacerbation. Plan — increased oxygen to four liters via nasal cannula, elevated head of bed to 45 degrees, notified provider with SBAR at 1535, stat chest X-ray and BNP ordered, anticipating possible diuretic administration pending lab and imaging results.

Narrative notes are the oldest and least structured format, consisting of chronological, free-text entries describing what happened during the shift or at a specific point in time. While narrative charting offers maximum flexibility, it is also the format most prone to disorganization, omissions, and irrelevant detail, which is precisely why most facilities have moved toward structured frameworks. However, narrative notes remain useful for documenting unusual events, patient incidents, detailed conversations with families or providers, and any situation where a structured format does not adequately capture the complexity of what occurred. When writing a narrative note, maintain chronological order, include the time of each entry, stick to objective and factual language, and avoid editorializing. A narrative entry might read: "At 2215 patient found on floor beside bed, call light within reach but not activated. Patient alert and oriented, states 'I was trying to get to the bathroom and my legs gave out.' Vital signs stable — BP 128/76, HR 82, RR 16, SpO2 97 percent on room air. Full neurological assessment performed, no focal deficits noted, pupils equal and reactive. Skin assessment reveals 3-centimeter abrasion to right elbow, superficial, minimal bleeding, cleansed with normal saline, adhesive bandage applied. Assisted back to bed with gait belt, two-person assist. Bed alarm reactivated, bed lowered to lowest position, call light placed within reach, patient instructed to use call light before attempting to ambulate. Provider notified at 2230, orders received for neurological checks every two hours for next eight hours and a morning CT head if any change in mental status. Patient's daughter called and informed of fall per patient's request." That narrative captures the event, the assessment, the interventions, the communication, and the follow-up plan in a way that would withstand scrutiny from any reviewer.

Regardless of which framework your facility uses, a few principles apply universally. Chart in real time whenever possible, because delays introduce memory errors and the legal record becomes less credible when notes are clustered at the end of a shift. Use objective language — document what you observed, measured, and did, not what you believe or suspect without supporting data. Avoid vague terms and quantify wherever you can: "large amount of drainage" means different things to different people, but "approximately 150 milliliters of serosanguineous drainage in the Jackson-Pratt over the past eight hours" means the same thing to everyone. Never alter a previous entry by deleting or overwriting — use a late entry or addendum with the current time, referencing the time of the original event, per your facility's policy. And always remember that the chart is a communication tool first: the nurse who reads your note at three in the morning during a change in condition should be able to understand exactly where the patient stood when you left.

8.2 The Daily Grind of Charting — I&O, the MAR, Flowsheets, and the Mistakes That Get Nurses in Trouble

Beyond the narrative and structured notes covered in the previous section, the majority of your charting time will actually go toward the routine, repetitive documentation that runs continuously through every shift: intake and output, the medication administration record, and assessment flowsheets. These are the entries that rarely feel dramatic, which is exactly why students underestimate how much they matter. A jury does not need a dramatic narrative note to determine whether a patient was adequately monitored — a gap in the I&O record or a missing flowsheet entry can be just as damaging as a poorly written paragraph.

Intake and output documentation tracks fluid balance, and its accuracy directly affects clinical decisions about hydration, diuretic dosing, kidney function, and heart failure management. Intake includes everything the patient consumes or receives: oral fluids, IV fluids, tube feedings, blood products, and even the fluid volume of medications given intravenously if your facility requires that level of detail. Output includes urine, emesis, drain output, wound drainage, diarrhea, and any other measurable fluid loss. The practical challenge is that this data accumulates throughout the shift from multiple sources, and the temptation is to estimate at the end rather than record as you go. Resist that temptation. Measure urine in a graduated container rather than eyeballing the collection bag, record oral intake using standard conversion measures your facility provides — an 8-ounce cup typically converts to approximately 240 milliliters — and document IV fluid volumes at the start and end of your shift plus any bag changes in between. When a patient is on strict I&O, meaning every measurable fluid is tracked, missing even one voiding or one cup of coffee can throw off a running total that a provider is using to make a diuretic dosing decision. If a patient refuses to use a urinal or void into a hat for collection, document that specifically rather than leaving the field blank, because a blank field is indistinguishable from a nurse who forgot to check.

The medication administration record, or MAR, is arguably the most legally scrutinized document in the chart, because it directly answers the question of whether the patient received what was ordered, when, and by whom. Most facilities now use electronic MARs integrated with barcode scanning, which automatically timestamps administration when you scan the patient and the medication. Your responsibility is to document immediately at the time of administration, not to batch several medications together and chart them all at once from memory twenty minutes later. If a medication is held, refused, or unavailable, you must document the reason using the specific codes or free-text explanation your system requires — "held, systolic blood pressure 88" or "refused, patient reports nausea, provider notified." An empty MAR entry for a scheduled medication is one of the fastest ways to trigger a medication error investigation, even if the medication was actually given, because the record shows no evidence that it was. PRN medications require an additional layer: document the reason for administration, the assessment that justified it, and — critically — the reassessment of effectiveness within the appropriate timeframe. Giving a PRN pain medication without later charting a pain reassessment leaves the chart unable to demonstrate that the intervention worked, which matters both clinically and legally.

Assessment flowsheets organize routine physical assessment findings into a grid format, typically with body systems listed down one side and time intervals across the top, allowing anyone reviewing the chart to quickly scan for trends. Completing a flowsheet efficiently means performing your assessment first, in full, and then translating your findings into the flowsheet's dropdown options or fields — never the reverse. Some flowsheets default to "within defined limits" or "normal" for every field unless changed, which creates a serious risk: if you do not actually assess a particular system and simply accept the default, you have effectively fabricated a normal finding. Every field you leave unchanged should reflect something you genuinely assessed and found to be normal, not a box you skipped. When you find an abnormal result, most electronic systems prompt for additional detail — use that space fully rather than selecting the abnormal option and moving on, because "abnormal" alone tells the next clinician nothing about what kind of abnormal you found.

Now consider the errors that appear again and again in real charts and in legal cases involving nursing documentation. Late entries are the most common. A late entry itself is not wrong — sometimes you cannot chart in the moment because you are actively managing an emergency — but an undisclosed late entry is a serious problem. The correction is straightforward: when charting after the fact, note the current time as the entry time, then within the body of the note write "late entry for [time of event]" and proceed to document what happened at that earlier time. This transparency protects you, because a reviewer who later notices a timestamp discrepancy will trust a clearly labeled late entry far more than an entry that silently misrepresents when it was written.

Vague language is the second recurring problem. A note that says "patient tolerated procedure well" tells a reviewer almost nothing — tolerated well according to what measure? Vital signs stable? No reported pain? No bleeding? The corrected version specifies: "patient's vital signs remained within baseline range throughout the procedure, denied pain greater than 2 out of 10, no bleeding noted at the site post-procedure." Similarly, "wound looks okay" should become "wound edges approximated, no drainage noted, surrounding skin without erythema or warmth." Specificity is not about writing longer notes for the sake of length; it is about ensuring that anyone reading the note six months from now, without having been in the room, can reconstruct exactly what you observed.

The third and most serious category is subjective opinion presented as objective fact. Writing "patient is drug-seeking" or "patient is non-compliant" or "family is difficult" inserts your personal judgment into a legal document in a way that can bias future care, and more importantly, it is rarely defensible because it describes your interpretation rather than an observable behavior. The corrected approach documents behavior without the label: instead of "patient is drug-seeking," write "patient has requested pain medication four times in the past two hours, rating pain consistently at 10 out of 10 despite receiving medication within the ordered interval each time; assessment reveals no observable signs of distress such as grimacing, guarding, or elevated vital signs during these requests." Instead of "family is difficult," write "patient's daughter has asked to speak with the charge nurse three times this shift regarding concerns about pain management; each concern was addressed and documented separately." This distinction — describing behavior versus assigning a label — is one of the most important shifts a nursing student can make in their documentation habits, because labels can follow a patient through their entire hospitalization and shape how subsequent staff approach their care, sometimes unfairly.

Charting defensively does not mean charting fearfully or padding notes with unnecessary detail. It means writing entries that are accurate, timely, specific, and objective, because a chart built on those four principles protects the patient by creating a reliable record of their care, and it protects you by demonstrating exactly what you did and why.

8.3 Surviving the Academic Paperwork Without Losing Your Weekend

Clinical documentation for patient care is only half of what nursing school demands. The other half is academic paperwork — care plans, concept maps, and clinical reflections — and this is the documentation that tends to consume entire weekends if you do not approach it strategically. The good news is that these assignments are not designed to torture you; they are designed to build the same clinical reasoning skills you are developing at the bedside, just in a slower, more deliberate format that gives your instructor visibility into your thought process. The bad news is that most students tackle them inefficiently, starting from a blank template and trying to write comprehensively about everything at once, which is exactly the approach that turns a two-hour assignment into a six-hour one.

Care plans exist to translate your assessment findings into an organized plan of nursing care, and the single most important skill within a care plan is writing an accurate nursing diagnosis, because everything else in the document flows from it. The standard structure for a nursing diagnosis statement follows the PES format: Problem, Etiology, and Signs and Symptoms. The Problem is the nursing diagnosis itself, selected from a standardized list such as NANDA International, phrased as the patient's actual or potential health issue — for example, "Impaired Gas Exchange" or "Risk for Infection." The Etiology is the "related to" component, identifying the underlying cause or contributing factor connected to that problem — related to alveolar-capillary membrane changes, related to invasive procedure, related to decreased mobility. The Signs and Symptoms component, sometimes called the "as evidenced by" portion, lists the specific objective and subjective data from your assessment that support the diagnosis — as evidenced by oxygen saturation of 89 percent on room air, crackles auscultated in bilateral lower lobes, and patient report of dyspnea on exertion. Put together, a complete nursing diagnosis reads: "Impaired Gas Exchange related to alveolar-capillary membrane changes as evidenced by oxygen saturation of 89 percent on room air, bilateral crackles in lower lung fields, and patient report of dyspnea on exertion." Notice that a risk diagnosis omits the signs and symptoms portion entirely, since by definition the problem has not yet occurred — a risk diagnosis is written simply as "Risk for Infection related to surgical incision and invasive IV access," because there is no evidence to cite for something that has not happened yet. Once your diagnosis is accurately written, the rest of the care plan — goals, interventions, and evaluation — should logically address that specific etiology, not the diagnosis in the abstract. If your etiology is decreased mobility, your interventions should target mobility, not generic respiratory care unrelated to that specific cause.

Concept maps ask you to visually connect a patient's diagnoses, lab values, medications, and nursing diagnoses in a way that demonstrates you understand how they relate to one another, rather than treating each piece of data as isolated. The efficient way to build one is to start with the patient's primary medical diagnosis in the center, then branch outward to the body systems it affects, the relevant lab values and their significance, the medications and why each one is prescribed for this specific patient, and finally your nursing diagnoses connected by lines showing which pieces of data support which diagnosis. Students who struggle with concept maps are usually trying to include everything from the chart rather than the data that actually tells the clinical story. Before you start drawing, ask yourself which five or six findings, if you had to explain this patient to a classmate in two minutes, actually matter — those are the elements that belong on your map, connected with clear, labeled relationships rather than a tangle of arrows.

Clinical reflections, sometimes called journals or self-evaluations, ask you to process what you experienced and what you learned, and they suffer most from students treating them as an afterthought completed hastily the night before submission. A strong reflection follows a simple structure: briefly describe a specific situation from your shift, rather than summarizing the entire day; explain your emotional and clinical response to that situation honestly; identify what you learned or what you would do differently; and connect that learning to a specific course objective or nursing concept. A reflection about your first time recognizing a deteriorating patient carries far more depth and earns more credit than a generic paragraph about "learning a lot today." Write these while the shift is still fresh, ideally the same evening, because the specific details that make a reflection meaningful fade quickly, and a reflection written three days later tends to be vague for the same reason a late clinical note is often vague — memory degrades faster than students expect.

The broader strategy for all of this academic paperwork is the same: do the thinking work during clinical, not after. Jot notes on your brain sheet about a moment worth reflecting on, a lab value connected to a diagnosis for your concept map, or the specific etiology behind a problem you assessed, while the information is fresh and in front of you. Arrive home with raw material rather than a blank page, and the writing itself becomes a matter of organizing what you already captured rather than reconstructing an entire shift from memory. This habit alone will save you more hours across a nursing program than almost any other time-management strategy available to you.

With both patient documentation and academic paperwork now covered, the next chapter turns to the moments when everything you have learned so far — assessment, labs, medications, procedures, and clear communication — converges under pressure: recognizing and responding to a patient in crisis.

Chapter 9 — Emergencies and Rapid Response

9.1 Learning to See Trouble Before It Becomes an Emergency

Every experienced nurse has a version of the same story: a patient who seemed fine, then somehow was not, and the nurse who caught it early enough to change the outcome describes a feeling that is hard to name precisely — a sense that something was off before any single number confirmed it. Students often assume this instinct is unteachable, a kind of intuition that only comes with years at the bedside. In truth, it is pattern recognition, and pattern recognition can be taught deliberately, long before you have logged those years. Patients almost never crash without warning. They deteriorate along a trajectory, and that trajectory leaves footprints in their vital signs, their mental status, and their lab values hours before the situation becomes a code. Learning to read those footprints is the single most valuable clinical skill you can build during nursing school, because it is the skill that turns a nurse into the person who prevents the emergency rather than the person who responds to one.

Mental status change is often the earliest and most reliable indicator that something is going wrong, and it is also the sign most frequently dismissed by inexperienced clinicians because it can look like something else — fatigue, medication effect, or simply an older patient having "an off day." Do not accept that framing without investigation. A patient who was oriented and conversational at your morning assessment but is now vague, slow to respond, or answering questions inconsistently has changed, and that change deserves your full attention regardless of how it can be explained away. Early confusion or restlessness is frequently the body's response to inadequate oxygen delivery to the brain, whether from hypoxemia, hypotension, sepsis, or a metabolic derangement, and the brain often shows distress before other organs do because it is exquisitely sensitive to perfusion and oxygenation. Watch for subtler cues too: a patient who normally makes eye contact and tracks the conversation but now seems to drift mid-sentence, a patient who becomes unusually agitated or unusually withdrawn compared to their baseline, or a patient who simply "doesn't seem like themselves" according to family at the bedside — family members often notice this shift before it shows up on any monitor, and their observation is clinical data, not just a passing comment.

Respiratory distress is the second major category, and it announces itself in ways that go well beyond a raw respiratory rate. Watch the mechanics of breathing itself: is the patient using accessory muscles in the neck and shoulders to pull air in, a sign that normal breathing is no longer adequate? Are they positioning themselves upright or leaning forward, instinctively trying to maximize lung expansion? Can they complete a full sentence, or are they pausing every few words to breathe? A patient speaking in two- or three-word fragments is telling you something urgent regardless of what the pulse oximeter reads at that exact second. Nasal flaring, grunting with exhalation, and visible retractions between the ribs are all signs your assessment training should catch quickly, and any of them warrants immediate escalation of your evaluation, not a plan to recheck in thirty minutes. Pay attention also to color — cyanosis around the lips or under the nail beds is a late and serious sign, meaning the compensatory mechanisms have already been overwhelmed by the time you see it, so waiting for cyanosis to appear before acting means you have already lost valuable time.

Hemodynamic instability is the third pillar, and it requires you to think in trends rather than isolated numbers. A blood pressure of

100/60 might be entirely unremarkable for one patient and a serious red flag for another whose baseline runs 150/90. This is why reviewing prior vital signs before you take a new set matters so much — you are not just collecting a number, you are placing it on a trajectory. A heart rate that has climbed from 78 to 92 to 108 across three consecutive checks is a trend worth flagging even if 108 alone would not alarm you in isolation, because the direction of change often matters more than the single value. Narrowing pulse pressure, cool and clammy extremities, delayed capillary refill, and diminishing urine output are all signs that the body is compensating for inadequate perfusion by shunting blood away from the periphery and kidneys to protect the brain and heart — and compensation, by definition, means the situation is already serious even though the blood pressure itself may still look acceptable on paper. This is one of the most important lessons a student can absorb: a "normal" blood pressure in a compensating patient can be dangerously misleading, and the surrounding signs often reveal the truth before the blood pressure number does.

Abnormal lab trends complete the picture, and the emphasis again falls on trend rather than isolated result. A rising white blood cell count alongside a climbing lactate level suggests worsening infection or early sepsis. A falling hemoglobin across serial draws points toward ongoing blood loss even when a single value might still fall within a broadly acceptable range. A steadily rising creatinine signals kidney function that is deteriorating in real time, often in response to inadequate perfusion elsewhere in the body. These trends rarely announce themselves loudly; they show up as small, incremental changes that are easy to miss if you are only glancing at the most recent result rather than comparing it against the several results before it.

Because integrating mental status, respiratory findings, hemodynamic data, and lab trends into a single coherent judgment can be difficult, especially for a student still building clinical experience, many hospitals now use structured early warning tools to help quantify urgency objectively. The Modified Early Warning Score, commonly abbreviated MEWS, is among the most widely used. It assigns points across several physiological parameters — respiratory rate, heart rate, systolic blood pressure, temperature, and level of consciousness — with higher point values assigned to readings further from normal in either direction. The individual scores are added together to produce a single composite number, and that number is compared against a facility-defined threshold that triggers escalation: a request for a repeat set of vitals sooner than scheduled, a call to the primary nurse or charge nurse, or in more urgent cases, activation of a rapid response team. The genuine value of a tool like MEWS is that it does not rely on subjective impression alone. A patient can look reasonably stable to an inexperienced eye while their MEWS score is already climbing into a range that demands immediate attention, and the score gives you an objective, defensible basis for escalating your concern even when you are still developing the clinical confidence to trust your own gut instinct. Learn how your facility calculates and uses its own version of this scoring system, because the specific point thresholds vary by institution, and knowing your unit's protocol means you will recognize exactly when a trending score requires you to act rather than simply observe.

The deeper lesson underlying all of this is that deterioration is rarely sudden. It is a story that unfolds gradually, told through small changes that are easy to dismiss individually but unmistakable once you learn to read them together. Developing that pattern recognition early, and pairing it with the objective backup of tools like MEWS, is what allows a nursing student to become the person in the room who notices trouble forming — long before it becomes the code that everyone remembers.

9.2 What to Actually Do When the Room Fills With People

The first time you witness a rapid response or a code blue, the sensation is disorienting. Within seconds, a quiet patient room transforms into a crowded space full of people moving with purpose, equipment appearing from nowhere, and a level of controlled urgency that feels like nothing else in nursing school. Most students freeze during their first exposure, not because they lack knowledge, but because nobody explained the choreography beforehand — where to stand, what role a student is expected to play, and what absolutely must be left to trained responders. Understanding that choreography in advance transforms the experience from paralyzing to purposeful, even if your role in the first several codes you witness is primarily to observe and assist at the margins.

Your first responsibility, the moment you recognize a patient is not right, is triggering the response system itself. Every hospital has a mechanism for this — a code button in the room, a specific phone number, or a call to the operator using standardized language like "rapid response, room 412" or "code blue, room 412." If you are the first person to notice a patient unresponsive, not breathing normally, or without a pulse, calling for help is your immediate action, before you do anything else, because a response team activated thirty seconds sooner can meaningfully change outcomes in situations like cardiac arrest. While waiting for the team to arrive, if you are trained and certified in Basic Life Support, and the patient is unresponsive without a pulse, begin chest compressions immediately — high-quality compressions started early are one of the strongest predictors of survival in cardiac arrest, and every second without them measurably lowers the odds. If you are not yet certified or the scenario does not call for compressions, stay with the patient, continue monitoring, and prepare to communicate clearly with the responding team the moment they arrive.

Once the response team is in the room, your position shifts, and this is where knowing your place prevents you from becoming an obstacle during a critical moment. As a student, position yourself against the wall or in a corner of the room where you have a clear view but are not in the direct pathway of the code team, the crash cart, or the bed itself. The room will fill quickly with a defined set of roles: someone leading the code and calling out orders, someone performing compressions, someone managing the airway, someone recording events on a code sheet, someone pushing medications, and often a pharmacist calculating doses. Each of these roles is typically filled by a licensed nurse, respiratory therapist, or physician who has been trained and credentialed specifically for that function. Your role is not to insert yourself into any of these positions uninvited. What you can do, and what experienced staff genuinely appreciate, is making yourself quietly useful at the edges: fetching supplies when someone calls out for them, helping clear the hallway or move furniture out of the way, assisting with communication if a family member is present and needs to be guided out of the room calmly, or holding open a door. If someone directs you to do something specific — hand them a piece of equipment, help reposition the patient, apply pressure somewhere — follow that instruction promptly and precisely, because during a code, instructions are not suggestions.

There are things you should never touch or attempt unsupervised during an active emergency, and knowing this boundary is as important as knowing how to help. Do not administer any emergency medication unless you are specifically directed to do so by a supervising nurse or provider who remains present and accountable for that action, and even then, only within the scope your program has authorized. Do not operate the defibrillator. Do not adjust ventilator or airway equipment. Do not make independent decisions about interventions during an active code — this is a moment for following the lead of the code team, not for initiative outside your training. It can feel uncomfortable to stand back while chaos unfolds around you, especially if you feel eager to help more directly, but restraint in this specific context is not passivity; it is exactly what a well-functioning code team needs from every person in the room who is not assigned a specific task.

Familiarizing yourself with the crash cart before you ever need it will make you significantly more useful when a real emergency happens. Most crash carts are organized in a standardized drawer system: airway equipment in one drawer, IV supplies and fluids in another, cardiac medications in another, and a defibrillator mounted on top or attached to the side. Take five minutes early in a clinical rotation to open the drawers on your unit's crash cart with a staff nurse and simply look. Knowing that epinephrine and atropine live in the medication drawer, that the ambu bag and oral airways sit in the airway drawer, and where the backboard is stored means that if someone shouts for a specific item during an emergency, you can locate and retrieve it in seconds rather than searching helplessly while precious time passes. This single piece of preparation does more to build genuine confidence for code situations than almost anything else available to a student.

9.3 After the Emergency Ends: Documentation, Debriefing, and the Scenarios You Are Most Likely to See

When a code or rapid response concludes, the work is not finished, even though the adrenaline in the room begins to fade. Documentation of the event must be completed thoroughly and promptly, typically using a specific code documentation form that captures the timeline in precise detail: the time the patient was found in distress, the time the response was called, the time compressions began if applicable, each medication given and at what time, each rhythm check and its result, any defibrillation attempts and their timing, and the ultimate outcome and disposition of the patient. As a student, you will likely not be the primary documenter during the event itself, but you may be asked to help verify times or details afterward, and understanding how detailed and time-specific this documentation must be reinforces why paying close attention throughout the event — even from your position along the wall — matters. If you personally performed compressions or assisted directly, you will typically complete your own brief documentation of your role and actions, and doing so accurately and promptly, while your memory of the sequence is still fresh, protects both the record and your own clarity about what occurred.

Most units conduct some form of debriefing after a significant emergency, and this practice serves two distinct but equally important purposes. Clinically, a debrief allows the team to review what happened, identify what went well, and honestly discuss what could have gone more smoothly — whether that means faster equipment access, clearer role assignment, or communication gaps during the event. These conversations are not about assigning blame; they are how teams improve their response for the next emergency, and participating thoughtfully, even as a student observer, teaches you an enormous amount about real-time crisis management that no textbook can replicate. The second purpose is emotional. Witnessing a code, especially your first one, or one with a difficult outcome, can be genuinely distressing, and it is normal to feel shaken afterward regardless of how composed you appeared in the room. Do not dismiss that reaction or feel that you need to hide it. Talk to your instructor, your assigned nurse, or a counselor if your program offers one. Processing what you witnessed is not a sign of weakness — it is part of building sustainable resilience for a career that will include more moments like this one, and nurses who suppress these reactions rather than processing them tend to struggle more, not less, over the course of a long career.

Beyond cardiac arrest, several other emergency scenarios appear regularly enough during clinical rotations that you should have an immediate action sequence ready for each. Anaphylaxis presents with rapid onset of symptoms following exposure to an allergen — medication, food, latex, or a contrast dye — and may include hives, facial or airway swelling, wheezing, difficulty breathing, and a sudden drop in blood pressure. The immediate priorities are stopping the causative exposure if it is still ongoing, such as halting an infusion, calling for help immediately, administering epinephrine per protocol or provider order as the first-line treatment, positioning the patient to support breathing, and preparing for oxygen administration and further airway support if swelling progresses.

Hypoglycemia requires fast recognition because symptoms can escalate quickly to altered consciousness. Watch for shakiness, diaphoresis, confusion, irritability, or a rapid heart rate in any patient receiving insulin or oral hypoglycemic agents. Confirm with a fingerstick glucose immediately. If the patient is conscious and able to swallow safely, give fifteen to twenty grams of fast-acting oral glucose — juice, glucose tablets, or gel — and recheck the blood sugar in fifteen minutes, repeating the treatment if it remains low. If the patient is unconscious or unable to safely swallow, intravenous dextrose or intramuscular glucagon becomes necessary, and this requires immediate provider notification and often falls outside independent student action, meaning your role is to recognize the situation and call for help without delay.

Seizures call for a response focused entirely on protection rather than restraint. Do not attempt to hold the patient down or place anything in their mouth, both of which are outdated practices that can cause injury. Instead, protect the patient's head, clear the immediate area of hazards, turn them onto their side if possible once the active seizure activity allows it to protect the airway from secretions, and time the duration of the seizure, because a seizure lasting longer than five minutes constitutes status epilepticus and requires emergency intervention. After the seizure ends, assess airway, breathing, and level of consciousness, and stay with the patient through the postictal period, during which confusion and fatigue are expected but should gradually improve.

Falls require immediate assessment before any attempt to move the patient. Do not rush to lift a patient who has fallen without first checking for injury, particularly head trauma or suspected fracture. Assess level of consciousness, check for obvious deformity or bleeding, and take a full set of vital signs before assisting the patient up, using appropriate assistive devices and additional staff as needed. Any fall involving head impact, loss of consciousness, or a patient on anticoagulant therapy warrants heightened concern for internal bleeding and typically triggers a neurological monitoring protocol and possible imaging.

Acute chest pain demands rapid, structured evaluation given the possibility of an evolving cardiac event. Obtain a full set of vital signs immediately, apply oxygen if the patient is hypoxic, and ensure a twelve-lead electrocardiogram is obtained promptly, as most facilities have a target of within ten minutes for patients presenting with chest pain. Ask about the character, location, radiation, and severity of the pain, and notify the provider immediately while preparing for potential orders including aspirin, nitroglycerin, and further cardiac workup, all while continuing to monitor for any change in hemodynamic stability.

Across every one of these scenarios, the underlying skill is the same one this entire chapter has built toward: recognizing that something is wrong quickly, calling for help without hesitation, and taking the specific, appropriate first action while more definitive care arrives. None of these situations require you to manage the full emergency alone, and none of them should. What they require is exactly what you now have — a clear sequence to follow so that fear does not fill the space where action should be. That same clarity and composure under pressure carries directly into the next chapter, where the focus shifts from clinical crisis to the communication skills that hold a care team together, in emergencies and in every ordinary moment in between.

Chapter 10 — Communication That Builds Trust

10.1 Talking With Patients Like a Nurse, Not Like a Script

Every nursing student learns therapeutic communication techniques early in their program, usually through role-play scenarios in a skills lab that feel stiff and artificial. You practice saying "I hear that you're frustrated" to a classmate pretending to be upset, and it sounds rehearsed because it is rehearsed. Then you arrive on a real clinical floor, face an actual patient who is scared, in pain, or simply exhausted by the indignities of being hospitalized, and the scripted phrases you memorized suddenly feel wrong in your mouth. This is one of the most common and most fixable struggles students face: the gap between knowing therapeutic communication techniques academically and using them naturally, in a way that sounds like you rather than a textbook. Closing that gap is less about memorizing new phrases and more about understanding the purpose behind each technique deeply enough that you can adapt it to the actual human being in front of you.

Active listening is the foundation everything else builds on, and it is far harder than it sounds, especially when you are managing a full assignment and thinking about your next task while trying to be present with a patient. Genuine active listening means giving the patient your full attention rather than formulating your next question while they are still talking. It means noticing not just their words but their tone, their pace, and what they are not saying. A patient who says "I'm fine, just tired" while avoiding eye contact and picking at their blanket is communicating something beyond the literal words, and a nurse who only registers "fine" misses the actual message. Practically, active listening looks like sitting down when time allows rather than hovering in the doorway, maintaining appropriate eye contact, minimizing interruptions, and resisting the urge to jump immediately to problem-solving before the patient has finished expressing what is actually bothering them. Students often want to fix things quickly, which is a natural instinct, but sometimes a patient needs to feel heard before they need a solution, and rushing past that step can leave them feeling processed rather than cared for.

Open-ended questions are the tool that invites patients to actually talk, rather than simply confirming or denying something you have already assumed. The difference between "Are you in pain?" and "Can you tell me more about what you're feeling right now?" is enormous. The first question can be answered with a single word and often produces an inaccurate picture, because patients frequently minimize or misjudge their own pain when asked a yes-or-no question under pressure. The second question opens space for the patient to describe location, quality, triggers, and impact in their own words, giving you far richer clinical information. This applies well beyond pain assessment. Instead of asking a preoperative patient "Are you nervous about the surgery?" — which most people will reflexively answer "no" to avoid appearing weak — try "What's going through your mind as you think about tomorrow?" The shift from closed to open questions is a small linguistic change that produces a dramatically different quality of conversation, and it becomes natural with repetition far faster than students expect.

Reflection, as a communication technique, means restating or paraphrasing what the patient has expressed, which serves two purposes at once: it confirms to the patient that you have actually understood them, and it often helps the patient hear their own concern articulated back, which can lead them to elaborate further or arrive at clarity they did not have before speaking. If a patient says "I just don't know how I'm going to manage at home with this colostomy bag, my husband already does so much," a reflective response might be "It sounds like you're worried about becoming another burden for your husband." This is not simply repeating their words back mechanically — it is identifying the emotional core of what they said and naming it, which invites deeper conversation rather than shutting it down. Reflection feels awkward the first several times you try it, because it requires a kind of vulnerability in naming someone else's feelings out loud, but patients rarely experience it as awkward. They experience it as being truly heard, often for the first time since their admission.

Validation goes a step further than reflection by explicitly acknowledging that a patient's feelings, given their circumstances, make sense — without necessarily agreeing with their interpretation of events or their proposed course of action. A patient who is furious about a delayed test result is entitled to that frustration, and validating it might sound like "Waiting for answers when you don't feel well is genuinely hard, and it makes complete sense that the delay is frustrating you." This differs from simply appeasing the patient or promising something you cannot deliver. You can validate a feeling while still explaining a reality the patient may not want to hear, and in fact, patients tend to accept difficult information more readily once they feel their frustration has been acknowledged rather than dismissed or argued with.

These techniques matter most, and are hardest to execute, with the patients who challenge you emotionally: those who are anxious, confused, or outright uncooperative. With an anxious patient, resist the instinct to reassure prematurely with phrases like "everything will be fine," which can feel dismissive if the patient does not yet believe it and undermines your credibility if things do not, in fact, turn out fine. Instead, acknowledge the anxiety directly, offer concrete information where you have it, and stay present rather than rushing out of the room the moment the conversation becomes uncomfortable. With a confused or disoriented patient, therapeutic communication shifts toward simplicity, patience, and reorientation rather than complex explanation. Speak slowly, use short sentences, reintroduce yourself and explain where they are without assuming they remember from your last interaction, and avoid arguing with confused statements, since correcting a disoriented patient's false beliefs rarely produces clarity and often produces agitation instead; redirecting gently tends to work better than confronting directly. With an uncooperative or hostile patient, the instinct to become defensive or to match their tone must be actively resisted. Underneath most hostility in a hospital setting is fear, pain, loss of control, or a previous negative healthcare experience, and staying calm, setting clear and respectful boundaries, and avoiding taking the behavior personally will de-escalate far more situations than a defensive response ever will.

Cultural sensitivity and health literacy considerations run underneath every one of these interactions and shape how effectively your communication actually lands. Patients bring vastly different beliefs about illness, family involvement in care decisions, eye contact, physical touch, and end-of-life preferences, and assuming your own cultural framework is universal is one of the fastest ways to unintentionally alienate a patient or their family. Ask rather than assume — a simple question like "Is there anyone you'd like included in these conversations about your care?" respects family structures that vary widely without requiring you to have memorized every cultural norm in advance. Health literacy is a related but distinct consideration: a patient's education level, primary language, and prior exposure to the healthcare system all affect how much of your explanation they actually absorb, regardless of how clearly you think you explained it. Avoid medical jargon by default, and when you must use a clinical term, define it in plain language immediately afterward. Ask patients to explain information back to you in their own words — sometimes called the teach-back method — rather than simply asking "Does that make sense?" which nearly every patient will answer yes to regardless of actual comprehension, either from politeness or embarrassment.

None of this becomes natural overnight. The scripted phrases from your skills lab are a starting scaffold, not a final performance, and the goal is to internalize the underlying principles deeply enough that your own words, in your own voice, begin to carry them automatically. That shift — from reciting technique to genuinely communicating — is what patients notice immediately, whether or not they could ever name what changed.

10.2 Calling the Provider at 2 AM Without Losing Your Nerve

There is a specific kind of dread that builds in a new nurse's chest at the thought of calling a physician in the middle of the night. The fear is rarely about the clinical content — you know your patient, you have the numbers, you understand the situation. The fear is about how the call itself will go: will you sound scattered, will you leave out something important, will the provider be short with you, will you freeze halfway through and forget what you were calling about in the first place. The antidote to that fear is not confidence you have to manufacture from nowhere. It is structure, and SBAR is the structure that turns a nervous, rambling phone call into a professional exchange that gets your patient what they need.

Before you dial, prepare. Have the patient's chart open, know their current vital signs and how they compare to baseline, know their allergies, know what medications they are currently receiving, and have a specific ask ready before the provider picks up. Walking into the call without a clear request is how conversations drift and how important details get lost. Once you have the provider on the line, introduce yourself clearly — your name, your role, the unit, and the patient's name and room number — and then move directly into the framework. Situation states what is happening right now, in one or two sentences. Background gives the essential context the provider needs to interpret that situation correctly. Assessment shares your clinical read of what is going on. Recommendation states specifically what you want: an order, a bedside evaluation, a lab, anything concrete.

Consider a realistic 2 AM scenario. A postoperative patient's blood pressure has been trending down over the last hour, and you need to call. You might open with, "This is Jordan, RN, calling from 4 West about your patient in room 218, Mr. Alvarez." Situation: "His blood pressure has dropped from 128/78 at midnight to 92/58 just now, and he's reporting increased pain at his surgical site." Background: "He's postoperative day one from a bowel resection, his hemoglobin this morning was 10.1, and he received his last dose of oxycodone about ninety minutes ago." Assessment: "He's pale, his heart rate has climbed to 104, and I'm concerned about either bleeding or inadequate volume." Recommendation: "I'd like to request a stat hemoglobin and hematocrit, and I think he needs to be evaluated at the bedside — would you like me to start a fluid bolus in the meantime?" That entire exchange takes under a minute to deliver, and it gives the provider everything they need to make a decision quickly, at an hour when nobody has patience for a disorganized story.

Requesting a new medication order follows the same logic, just with a slightly different recommendation. If your patient's pain is inadequately controlled on their current regimen, your SBAR might state the situation as persistent pain despite scheduled medication, background as the current orders and timing of the last dose, assessment as your evaluation that the current regimen appears insufficient for this patient's needs, and recommendation as a specific request — perhaps an increased dose, a different medication, or the addition of a PRN option. Coming to the provider with a specific, reasonable recommendation rather than simply reporting a problem and waiting to be told what to do demonstrates clinical thinking, and most providers respond well to nurses who bring solutions rather than only concerns.

Sometimes the first response you receive is inadequate, and this is where many students, especially as beginners, back down too quickly. If you call about a deteriorating patient and the provider says something like "just keep an eye on it and call me if it gets worse," but your clinical judgment tells you the situation is already concerning enough to warrant more, you are entitled — and expected — to escalate. This does not mean arguing or being combative. It means restating your concern with additional clarity: "I understand, but I want to make sure I'm communicating the urgency here — his blood pressure has dropped twenty points in an hour and he's tachycardic, and I'm not comfortable just monitoring without further evaluation. Can we talk about what specific parameters would prompt you to come see him, or should I contact the charge nurse or resident to get another set of eyes on him?" If the response remains unsatisfactory and your instinct still says something is wrong, the chain of command exists precisely for this situation — notify your charge nurse, your instructor, or the nursing supervisor, and do not feel that going up the chain reflects poorly on you. It reflects exactly the kind of patient advocacy nursing licensure exists to protect.

Handoff communication between shifts deserves the same structured attention, because this is the moment where errors and omissions most commonly slip through the cracks of patient care. A thorough handoff, often using SBAR or a similar structured format like I-PASS, should include the patient's diagnosis and reason for admission, any changes in condition during your shift, pending tasks or results, code status, and anything the oncoming nurse specifically needs to watch for. Resist the temptation to rush through handoff because you are eager to leave — the ninety seconds you save by skipping a detail can cost the incoming nurse, and the patient, far more than that later in the shift. Whenever possible, conduct handoff at the bedside, which allows both nurses to visually confirm the patient's status together and gives the patient an opportunity to correct or add information. This practice has become increasingly standard because it catches discrepancies that a hallway report alone would miss entirely.

10.3 The Conversations Nobody Practices in Skills Lab

Some of the hardest communication moments in nursing have nothing to do with clinical data at all, and nursing programs rarely give students a script for them, because there genuinely is no perfect script. What exists instead is a set of principles that can guide you through delivering bad news, defusing an agitated situation, and protecting yourself from disrespect within your own care team — three categories of conversation that every nurse eventually faces and that no amount of pharmacology knowledge prepares you for.

Delivering serious news to a family is usually not a task assigned to a student nurse directly — that responsibility typically belongs to the physician or provider — but you will frequently be present for these conversations, and you will absolutely be the person families turn to afterward with questions, emotions, and disbelief. Your role in these moments is not to soften the news or offer false reassurance, but to be a steady, honest presence. If a family asks you directly whether their loved one is going to be okay and the situation is genuinely uncertain, avoid promising an outcome you cannot guarantee. A response like "I know this is incredibly frightening, and I wish I had a clearer answer for you. What I can tell you is what the team is doing right now, and I will make sure you're updated as soon as we know more" is honest without being cold, and it keeps the family informed without overstepping into territory that belongs to the provider. Sit with families in their grief rather than rushing to fill silence with words. Sometimes your presence in the room, simply staying rather than leaving because the moment feels uncomfortable, communicates more compassion than anything you could say.

De-escalating an agitated patient requires managing your own physiological response as much as theirs. Keep your voice low and even, even if theirs is raised. Maintain a non-threatening body posture — avoid crossing your arms, standing directly in front of an exit blocking their path, or standing too close. Give the patient space to express their frustration without interrupting them, because interruption often escalates agitation rather than calming it. Once they have expressed the core of their frustration, acknowledge it specifically rather than generically: "You've been waiting almost two hours for your pain medication and nobody has explained why, and that's genuinely unacceptable — let me find out what happened." If the situation continues to escalate despite your efforts, know your facility's protocol for requesting additional support, whether that is calling for a charge nurse, security, or a behavioral response team, and never feel that requesting help in an unsafe situation reflects a personal failure. Your physical safety is not negotiable, and no amount of therapeutic communication training obligates you to remain in a genuinely dangerous situation.

Lateral incivility — the sometimes-discussed but rarely-addressed phenomenon of nurses being unkind to other nurses, including students — deserves direct acknowledgment, because it happens more often than nursing programs like to admit, and students frequently absorb it silently, assuming it is simply part of paying their dues. It is not something you have to accept. If a nurse speaks to you dismissively, excludes you from learning opportunities out of apparent irritation, or makes comments that undermine your confidence in front of patients or staff, a calm, direct response is appropriate: "I want to learn from you, and I'd appreciate it if we could communicate more directly when something isn't going well." If the behavior continues or escalates, involve your clinical instructor, who exists specifically to advocate for students in situations exactly like this one. You are not required to simply endure disrespect as the price of an education, and naming the behavior clearly, without hostility, is often the fastest way to change it.

All of this — the difficult conversations, the emotional weight of witnessing suffering, the accumulated stress of high-stakes decision-making — takes a genuine toll, and pretending otherwise does nursing students no favors. Build small, sustainable habits for processing what you experience: talk honestly with classmates who understand the specific pressures of clinical rotations, use your program's counseling resources if the weight of a particular shift lingers, and give yourself permission to feel affected by hard days rather than performing toughness you do not actually feel. The nurses who last decades in this profession are rarely the ones who never let anything touch them emotionally. They are the ones who found sustainable ways to process what they carry, shift after shift, so that compassion for patients never came at the total expense of compassion for themselves.

You now have the clinical knowledge, the procedural skills, and the communication tools that carry a nursing student from uncertain to genuinely capable at the bedside. What remains is bringing it all together — and that is exactly where the conclusion picks up.

Conclusion: You Are Ready for the Bedside

Think back to the introduction of this book, to that moment of standing frozen at the bedside while a question hangs in the air and your mind goes blank. If you have made it this far, that image should feel different to you now than it did on page one. Not because the pressure of clinical rotations has disappeared, and not because you will never again feel unsure of yourself in front of a patient or an instructor. It feels different because you now have something you did not have before: a complete, interconnected system for approaching every shift, and the understanding of how each piece of that system supports every other piece.

Consider how the ten chapters actually fit together, because the connections matter more than any single chapter on its own. You learned that clinical competence starts before you ever touch the unit floor, in the quiet discipline of reviewing a chart and building a worksheet the night before. That preparation feeds directly into your assessment skills, because a nurse who understands the patient's diagnosis walks into a head-to-toe assessment already knowing what to expect and what would represent a meaningful change. Your assessment findings only become useful once you can interpret them, which is why the lab values chapter exists — a heart rate of 110 means something different once you know the potassium is 2.9, and a BUN and creatinine climbing together tell a story that a single number never could on its own. That interpretation directly shapes medication safety, because understanding why a drug was prescribed and what to monitor before, during, and after administration depends entirely on knowing your patient's clinical picture, not just the order on the MAR. Medication knowledge extends naturally into IV therapy and the procedures chapter, where the calculations and safety checks you practiced on paper become the physical skills you perform with your hands. Every assessment, every medication, every procedure then has to be captured accurately in documentation, because a wound cared for perfectly but charted vaguely creates exactly the kind of gap that puts patients and licenses at risk. And all of that groundwork — assessment, interpretation, safe administration, documentation — becomes the foundation you stand on when a patient starts to deteriorate, because recognizing early warning signs is only possible when you already know what normal looks like for that specific person. Finally, none of it functions in isolation from the people around you. The communication skills in the final chapter are what allow you to advocate for your patient with a provider at 2 AM, hand off a shift without losing critical details, and hold yourself together through the emotional weight this profession inevitably asks you to carry.

This is the loop worth remembering: preparation enables assessment, assessment enables interpretation, interpretation enables safe intervention, intervention requires accurate documentation, documentation supports early recognition of deterioration, and communication ties every one of those pieces to the team around you. None of these skills exist as isolated facts to memorize for an exam. They are a single, continuous system, and you now own that system. Competence built one careful step at a time is what generates real confidence — not the fragile kind that collapses the first time something unexpected happens, but the durable kind that comes from knowing you have a reliable process to fall back on no matter what the shift throws at you.

Owning this system, though, means actually using it, and that starts with how you treat this book itself. Do not let it sit pristine on a shelf. Fold the corners of the pages you return to most. Underline the calculation formulas until the ink bleeds through. Tab the chapters by specialty so you can find what you need in seconds during a hectic shift. Bring it into your scrub pocket every single rotation, not just the first few weeks when everything feels unfamiliar, because pediatrics will ask different questions of you than medical-surgical did, and psychiatric clinical will demand a different kind of communication than the ICU. Revisit sections before you start each new specialty, because the muscle memory that felt automatic on one unit will need a quick refresher before it transfers cleanly to another. And let this book be the beginning of your professional habits, not the end of them. Join a nursing student organization if your school has one, because the connections and mentorship available there extend far beyond what any single guide can offer. Seek out a nurse you admire and ask if they would be willing to answer questions as you move through your program — most experienced nurses remember exactly what it felt like to be where you are now, and most are generous with their time when a student asks sincerely. Start building a professional portfolio of your clinical experiences, skills checked off, and reflections written along the way, because that record will serve you well when you are interviewing for your first position as a licensed nurse.

Here is the truth worth carrying with you as you close this book and head to your next shift: every nurse currently working confidently at the bedside once stood exactly where you are standing right now — unsure, a little frightened, quietly wondering whether they had what it took. The nurses who thrived were not the ones born with some innate gift the rest of us lack. They were the ones who prepared consistently, showed up even when they felt unready, and built their competence one shift at a time until confidence simply followed. You have that same path in front of you, and now you have a tool built specifically to walk it with you. You are ready for the bedside. Go show your patients what that readiness looks like.